ONE IN A MILLION

Brenda Baalham

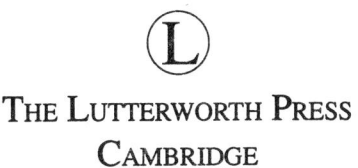

THE LUTTERWORTH PRESS
CAMBRIDGE

The Lutterworth Press
P.O. Box 60
Cambridge CB1 2NT

British Library Cataloguing in Publication Data
Baalham, Brenda
  One in a million.
  1. Care
  I. Title
  261.83

  ISBN 0-7188-2832-2

Printed in Great Britain by
The Guernsey Press Co. Ltd, Guernsey, Channel Islands.

Dedicated to my husband, Chris, for being 'one in a million'

CONTENTS

FOREWORD
by Jennifer Rees Larcombe

Whenever I open an envelope and find that the letter inside is from Brenda Baalham I know I am in for a treat. For some years now we have corresponded regularly and she has painted for me a vivid word-picture of her life as a disabled wife and mother. It is not surprising that someone who can make a letter so interesting is also capable of being a successful writer. When her articles began to appear in various magazines I found them just as perceptive and engrossing as her private letters.

It is always lovely to see anyone being a success in their lives, and I would certainly describe Brenda as a successful disabled person. It is possible to live a full, rich and useful life in spite of disabilities, but Brenda would probably be the first to admit that the secret of this ability lies in the devoted love of a carer. When her letters described how Chris had decided to give up his job so he could look after Brenda and their two young boys full-time I could not help thinking of the words of the Lord Jesus, 'the greatest love a person can have for his friends is to give up his life for them.' (John 15.13). I know from personal experience as a disabled mother just how much it costs someone to take on the full-time care of a handicapped person. It means giving up so many of the ordinary little things which most people take for granted. Yet this enormous sacrifice so often receives from the rest of the world inadequate recognition and practical support. This book is the story of one such carer - Chris himself - but it also includes the experiences of many more of these unsung heroes and gives very perceptive insights into their needs and emotional problems.

'What a 'One in a Million' Chris must be,' I thought as I read about him in Brenda's letters and when eventually I met him recently I knew he was certainly that. This is a book we have all been waiting to read for a very long time and I cannot recommend it highly enough.

ACKNOWLEDGEMENTS

I would like to thank all those in a professional or voluntary capacity who have helped to provide me with the background information necessary to complete this book. My gratitude, in particular, goes to: Sue Dawes, Joyce Miller, Marcia Start, Dr Richard Taylor and John Train.

I would also like to thank my family and friends for their encouragement and support during the last two years - in particular Christine Baalham and Janet Parratt who read my manuscript in its early stages and whose positive comments spurred me on, and Julia Burton-Jones and Benedicte Scholefield whose active support during the latter stages of the book was invaluable.

Much gratitude is also owed to the many carers who were willing to share their experiences with me, either personally or by letter. Space did not permit me to include all their stories but those which have been used serve to represent many carers in a variety of caring situations throughout the nation. I have altered all the carers' names in order to respect their privacy.

Most of all I would like to express my thanks for the gift of a word processor without which I could not have even begun!

Chapter 1
JUST ANOTHER OF THOSE DAYS!

The shrieks and yells coming from the garden had reached a peak. I don't know which was harder to endure: the noise, indicating that the children were running wild, or the periods of silence which followed when one was left to imagine what they were getting up to.

Timothy, then aged about 8, and Matthew, 4, had been left to their own devices for too long. They needed attention, that was obvious, but we were not able to give it to them. I was aware of the commotion and felt guilty that I was the cause of them being ignored. But I could do nothing about it and almost felt beyond caring anyway.

My husband, Chris, on the other hand, was being torn in two and didn't know which way to turn. The needs outside were desperate, but my needs took precedence.

Stomach upsets are never nice. When one has a home and family to care for they cause problems although most people are able to carry on, even if they feel awful. But in our household they have been a thing to fear for a number of years and something to be avoided at all costs. On this particular day, however, I had succumbed to a nasty tummy bug. I'd managed to keep going all day but by the time my husband came home at 5 o clock I'd come to the end of my tether.

Chris, assessing the situation, packed the children into the garden to play. They'd already been left to their own devices all day and were now tired and hungry but what else could he do?

He then managed to get me into the bedroom. I could now scarcely walk as each attack of vomiting left me stiffer and stiffer and before long I would be totally rigid. He eased me on to the bed and just had time to grab a bowl before the next bout. With me half-fainting and needing the bowl held, there was no chance to respond to the frenzied yells coming from outside.

As I recovered a little he sponged my face, gave me some water and laid me back on the bed. After clearing up the mess and applying disinfectant liberally everywhere he was able to put his head out of the back door and shout at the children in exasperation. This was not what they needed but he had no time for anything else and by now his nerves were frayed too.

It was time to get tea but he only got about half-way through the preparations when I had to summon him once more. By now I could not even raise myself to a sitting position and didn't dare remain lying down for too long.

But God knows how much we can take. We were far too preoccupied to have consciously prayed but, as Chris sat propping me up, waiting for the inevitable to happen, with the children yelling and the tea half made, help appeared in the form of a close friend. She offered to prop me up and hold the bowl and he was able to finish the tea and bring the children in to have it. Relative peace reigned once more and our friend quietly took her leave.

But the crisis was not over yet. Somehow he had to help me into the toilet, undress me and put me to bed. When every movement caused me to cry out in pain it was not an easy task ahead of him. The doctor would also have to be called. He would not be able to cure a stomach upset but I could not keep my pills down and so was getting worse by the minute. Chris would also have to get some tea for himself, clear away, put the boys to bed and, of course, be interrupted each time I was sick again!

During a breathing space before he embarked on these things he came in to see me. All he could do was to hold me in his arms and we both sobbed and sobbed. Most of the time we managed to cope with our circumstances but just sometimes they got on top of us and we wondered where it would all end. Our faith in a loving heavenly Father, who not only cared but was also in control, was stretched to the limit. But the crying did us both good and we were able to carry on.

Somehow, Chris got all the jobs done. The doctor came and gave me an injection to stop the vomiting and an injection of morphine for the pain and stiffness. Gradually I drifted into a wonderful, healing sleep and my husband had a chance to relax. Tomorrow things would be better.

It had just been another of those days - best forgotten about and put behind us. Such days were not too frequent but, nevertheless, frequent enough to cause Chris a sense of anxiety every evening as he peddled home from work on his bicycle.

At work he could put it all in the background for a few hours but each evening he had to face up to the fact that he never quite knew what he would find when he returned home. It would have been lovely to have been normal. Many of his colleagues returned home to relax in a chair as their dinner was being prepared. This would be followed by an evening of pleasing oneself whether it was going out with their wives, going to the pub, playing sport, or just watching television. Such lives were probably selfish and shallow and sometimes only existed in Chris's imagination but, nevertheless, they were something to be envied when his position was so different and when he had not had a break from this for years.

He might have been tempted to cycle in the opposite direction. In some ways running away would have been an easy solution for him and few would have blamed him for taking it.

Life had not always been so complicated. Our backgrounds, although totally separate, were very similar. We had both been brought up in a loving, secure and happy environment with very little to vex or perplex us. Our parents were Christians and neither of us had ever seriously rejected their teachings or doubted their faith. This did not of course make us Christians but their steady and faithful Christian example and prayers must have ultimately had an effect on us.

As we approached our mid-teens we were both challenged with the teachings of Christ and realised it was not enough to simply acknowledge in our heads all that we had been brought up to believe. We could no longer sit on the fence and say 'OK, I believe it all but so what?' We had to face the fact that Christ was calling us to do something about it.

We could reject Christ and carry on our lives quite independently from Him. Or we could acknowledge the fact that God wanted a relationship with us - a relationship that had been broken and marred by our own wilful natures - which could only be restored by accepting that God's Son, Jesus Christ had died for us on the cross. He had taken the punishment and blame which should have been ours. We could ask for forgiveness and invite God to take control of our lives from then on. We chose the latter course and from then on started on our Christian journey.

We went through all the normal ups and downs of teenage years: exams, finding the right career, leaving home and eventually finding the right marriage partner. All big events in our lives, at the time, and not to be belittled. But we firmly believed God to be in control and asked for His guidance to lead us through all these things. With hindsight, it is easy to see that He did and that we encountered very few major difficulties along the way.

Indeed, it all seemed so straightforward when we made our marriage vows to one another in the little Baptist Church in West London where we had met and worshipped together for about two years. It was a beautiful spring day, we were in love, we believed God had brought us together and we had the rest of our lives to love and serve Him and each other.

It was exciting too. We were about to make a new home and life in Cumbria. In 1974 it was a brand new county and the prospects before us seemed wonderful. It was easy to make those vows under such circumstances and I'm sure we meant every word.

The Minister gave us a Bible as was the custom of that church. In the front was a verse about 'standing firm in one spirit, with one mind striving side by side'. Such sentiments seemed a good goal to aim for. Little did we know what would befall us within the next two years and just how we would be called upon to stand firm together.

Had Chris, my husband, known what was in store he might well have been tempted to opt out. However, he promised to take me as his wife for better or worse, in sickness and in health and, although he never imagined that the negative aspects would appear in any long-term sense and however much he may have been tempted to cycle in the opposite direction when they did, this is what he has chosen to do. In doing so he has indeed become 'one in a million'.

He is not alone. There are over a million others like him in this country. He is not only one in a million but also one of a million! What do all these people have in common? They are the 'carers' in our society. They are those who look after an elderly, frail person or a severely sick or disabled one. They may not necessarily be a husband or wife. They could just as easily be a son or daughter or even a close friend. They may not be committed by their marriage vows as Chris is but the job they perform is just the same.

The job is full-time, often 24 hours a day, every day of the week, sometimes for years on end. 'I must always put his needs first. If he wants to go to bed and I'm watching the television - it goes off.' These words spoken by Mary, an acquaintance, sum up the typical attitude of a carer.

The majority of carers are aged between 40 and 60. 42% are over 60 and 8% are below 40. A growing number are in their teens or even younger!*

Caring for someone is often arduous, physical work. It not only involves keeping an eye on someone but also general housework and in many cases lifting, dealing with incontinence, helping with feeding, dressing, bathing and toileting. It is no wonder that 58% of carers suffer from some kind of health problem and that 16% suffer from back trouble and strain due to lifting and general exhaustion through lack of sleep and over-exertion. Up to 50% are said to be found at risk of psychiatric illness.

Most of those they care for will be elderly. About three quarters of those needing help will be physically handicapped and about 16% will suffer from both mental and physical problems. In addition to their caring role, many people will have other responsibilities too, giving up many hours a week in this way and also remaining in paid employment or having other dependants making demands on their time and energy.

Nevertheless, they carry on out of love and duty in a selfless, conscientious and tireless way. They perform often thankless and difficult tasks with very little complaint in their own ceaseless and quiet manner. They would probably be the last people to give themselves the name of 'carer' and yet this is what they are ... silent saints indeed! Although their work can be very tiring and stressful they often get very little help and can be very isolated. About one quarter have looked after the same person for more than 10 years and although most can manage an hour or two's break with help, many could never manage and never have managed a break even for as long as a day or two.

Carers don't say much about themselves. Because of the very nature of their occupation they can easily be passed by ... unheard of, unknown, unrecognised and as a result often sadly neglected. We know something of the heartache and problems involved in being a carer. We have learned through many years of experience. I say 'we' because in all these years we have 'striven side by side' and in many ways it is hard to separate the carer from the one who is being cared for.

All carers (not just my husband) are 'one in a million' but they are also only human. Maybe it is time to speak out on their behalf, not only making their existence and the problems they face known to others, so that they may receive help and support where necessary, but also, by way of personal testimony, sharing a common experience with them and offering words of encouragement and a hope in the love and care of the Lord Jesus Christ who is the ultimate solution to all our needs.

* = OPCS - 1985. General Household Survey in 1985 was asked by DHSS to include questions to identify people looking after a sick, disabled or elderly person and to provide national estimates of the numbers of such carers. The statistics found in this chapter (and anywhere else) come from a summary of this survey.

Chapter 2
TO BE OR NOT TO BE A CARER?...

... that is the question. It is the first question the potential carer needs to ask. Being a carer is not something one chooses like a career or hobby. It is brought about through circumstances, which one would never choose and which will vary for each and everyone of us. There are no hard and fast rules to follow but every person faced with the possibility of becoming a carer will need to decide whether they will actually be able to fulfil the role.

Decision-making is never easy, especially when they are big and far-reaching decisions that have to be made. For some the situation arises suddenly and unexpectedly, perhaps as the result of an accident, sudden illness or the birth of a handicapped child. When presented with such a sudden shock there is a feeling of numbness and one's mind and emotions are in a turmoil. It is very difficult to make any decision under such circumstances.

It would be very easy to make rash decisions and become a carer out of duty or for purely emotional reasons. So easy to say when dealing with a loved one: 'I'll care for them for the rest of my life' without really exploring the implications of such a statement. Care may be required for years or may be of the kind that one is unable, however willing, to give. Hasty decisions will only be regretted and if promises and commitments cannot be kept, guilt may well be the result.

Some people have no one to turn to. Friends and relatives may desert them or be so out of their depth or bowled over themselves that they are of little help. Even worse, some carers are unable to share the situation with the person they are caring for because they may be mentally disturbed, handicapped, confused, a child or perhaps just awkward, cantankerous or bitter.

Our situation was very different. My condition deteriorated slowly and gradually and we had years in which to come to terms with it. Any decisions Chris needed to make did not have to be made in haste or rashly. We had time to deal with our emotions and often our wounds were not raw.

Chris was fortunate in that he had a good relationship with me too. We have always been good friends and communicated easily and naturally over everything and, as my mind had not been affected he was able to talk about and share the decision-making with me.

We were also blessed in being surrounded by a loving, caring circle of friends and family who offered much in the way of practical help and support. They were loyal and faithful and without them we would have found it very difficult to cope.

All our decisions, throughout the years, have thus been able to be made within a good framework. How much worse for others who have few or even none of these things! Yet, with hindsight, I can see that even we had to make it on our own with God and that we felt very isolated at times. We felt like pioneers stepping out into a little known, almost unexplored area.

There is a great need for advice and support for potential carers and for carers themselves. More and more people are becoming aware of this need but I feel it is still a neglected area and one particularly misunderstood and poorly comprehended by Christians. This is very sad. It is marvellous that advice is becoming more widespread but when Christians have that 'little bit extra' to offer it's a pity more people aren't receiving Christian advice! Christians and non Christians alike can benefit from such help as long as it is wisely and prayerfully given and as long as the counsellor concerned has taken the time and trouble to gain some insight into the problems faced by the carer.

The Christian carer is not only presented with the problem of finding the most obvious natural solution but also of understanding what God wants. Thankfully He knows our needs and what is best for us and treats us all as individuals, and therefore it is obvious there is never going to be any cut and dried answer. Generally speaking though, we can be assured that He doesn't permit us to be tested beyond our endurance and that He does expect us to use our God-given common sense. He will guide if we are really willing to listen and be open to His voice, and not focus on ourselves all the time.

This is often easier said than done and this is where it could be so helpful to have other Christians around to listen and offer counsel and to pray both in helping a person to come to a decision and also in supporting them in it. At this stage people are so often confused and become very introverted so it is hard for them to see where they are being led. Some good solid support and advice would be so useful in answering the initial question as to whether to become a carer or not.

For some the decision is taken out of their hands. They may be physically or mentally unable to meet the demands that will be made upon them. Maybe some would be able to manage with a lot of statutory and voluntary help but it is just not available or adequate for them. Others may not be willing or able to cope with the self sacrifice it may entail. Maybe they have a job or career which they feel it is right to continue with and think alternative means to care for the loved one would be better. For some there are other members of the family to consider and it would not be wise or practical to neglect them for the one to be cared for. We can only do so much!

Take Pauline: She is a very loving, caring person and is obviously very fond of her family. When her mother became mentally ill and unable to live on her own anymore Pauline's first thought was to give up her job and have her mother live with her. She felt guilty at the thought of doing anything else. But after much careful thought and soul-searching she decided against this course of action. Recently divorced, with two young children, she had their needs as well as her own to consider. She needed the outlet of her career, at that moment in time, to help her cope. The children had already experienced upheaval and found the sudden change in a once very capable, active granny hard to understand. Her mother too didn't really want to live with them. She could not cope with the children either. So Pauline's mother went to a home. Pauline still cares for her - visiting, having her to stay and sorting her affairs out. Her mother is happy and has improved a lot. They are all coping with a difficult situation, whereas had Pauline become a carer it might have been disastrous for all concerned and caused far more harm.

There are many good and valid reasons for not becoming a carer. As long as we are not trying to run away from our responsibilities and are earnestly trying to come up with the best solution for all concerned there should be no need for feelings of guilt to creep in. Christian counsel and support is so useful not only in helping us to decide what is best but also in supporting us in the decision reached and helping prevent regrets.

There will be alternative courses available to the potential carer.

* The first stage is perhaps to consult the dependant, if possible, and see what they want.

* In some situations there may be other relatives or friends better suited to the task.

* Failing this the state can step in a variety of ways. Consulting one's doctor, who will be able to put you in touch with all the right statutory

bodies, is probably the most simple way of discovering what other arrangements can be made.

* Voluntary organisations can also be very useful and can often be used to fill in some of the gaps in the statutory system or those which friends and relatives are unable to perform.

There will be points for and against every course of action available. Nothing will be perfect. It is very important, before one finally decides that it is not right to become a carer, that every other option is explored fully. One's mind can then be put at rest about the ultimate decision made, knowing that it is the best one possible in the circumstances.

Chapter 3
WHATEVER NEXT?

The decision to be a carer has been made! But that is just the start. Where does one go from there? Every carer's situation is slightly different and the way forward will really depend on the individual needs and circumstances of those concerned.

It may all appear very confusing and frightening to the new carer but there do seem to be several basic courses to take and each one will need to be thought about carefully.

* For some it will only involve caring part-time and for a person or persons outside their immediate household. With help, the dependant can still manage to live apart from the carer. About 70% of all carers will be caring for someone in this sort of situation i.e. for someone outside their immediate household. Parents or friends are obviously the most common people to be cared for and most will be living alone.

* For others the person to be cared for may need a lot of attention and will need to become a part of the household. The most common group of carers in this category is a son or daughter caring for a parent (or parents).

* Many carers begin to care for someone who already lives in their home ... usually for a spouse (most commonly) or a child. About 30% of carers care for someone in the same household.

Whatever category one falls into, there will be so many areas to explore and investigate before any final decisions are taken as to the extent of care one is able to provide and whether it will be satisfactory.

* There will be other commitments which may need adapting or even relinquishing ... job, social activities, hobbies, church etc.

* The majority of carers will have other members of the family to consider. About one third of all carers have dependent children, in most cases in addition to the person they are looking after.

* Assistance from voluntary or statutory sources may be essential.
* Sometimes homes will need to be adapted.

The list is endless and probably has to be dealt with at a time when one is finding it difficult to think straight! But do take time to investigate it all fully and don't rush into anything.

There are several chapters at the back of this book devoted to the kind of help which may be available. Professional advice from a social worker or doctor can be very useful in helping one define one's role and also sorting out all the practical details. Remember also, voluntary bodies and friends have an important part to play too.

Caring is an ongoing thing. Conditions and circumstances never remain the same. Once a carer does not necessarily mean always a carer or always the same kind of carer. The situation will need reviewing from time to time.

* If the dependant's condition deteriorates, more caring will be required. This may or may not be possible.

* The carer himself may no longer be able to continue; perhaps because of age or ill health or other personal problems the strain may become too much.

* The dependant may improve and need less help.

* The dependant may need about the same amount of help but this may alter as circumstances or their condition change.

Both carer and dependant need to be flexible. Pauline's circumstances, two years on, have changed and she is re-thinking her role. Her mother is much improved. She can enjoy the grandchildren and her friends again. She visits Pauline frequently. Her bungalow has been rented during all this time. It does not seem likely that she will ever be well enough to return to it but, if her condition remains stable, she does not really need to remain in the nursing home either. Pauline and the children are more settled too. So now Pauline is considering selling her mother's house and her own and moving them all to a larger property with a 'granny' flat attached. If they do so her role will change. She will need to be at least a partial carer and keep a greater eye on her mother than when she was cared for in the nursing home. But perhaps circumstances are now right for her to make that change.

Our circumstances changed too, but for us they deteriorated rather than improved. For 10 years my husband was able to retain his career. I was able to cope with myself and the house reasonably well. I could drive and retained a degree of independence in this way. We were able to have two lovely children during the earlier stages of my disease and, although much of their care had to be given over to others, we coped. Had we not had practical support from friends, relatives and the Social Services Chris would have had to have given up his job years previously. But as the disease slowly and relentlessly pursued its course, we finally got to the point where some decisions and changes needed to be faced once more. The welfare of ourselves as well as that of the children needed careful consideration.

As I became increasingly and more rapidly disabled the support we had relied upon was no longer adequate. On a purely practical level we could have carried on in this way, I suppose. Instead, we stopped to consider our quality of life and found it lacking.

The children had been marvellous. The elder one could remember a time when Mummy was fairly independent and could do the cooking and cleaning and take him out in the car to visit friends or playschool and then school itself. He was aware of a lot of helpers who did the things Mummy couldn't manage and looked after him and played with him a lot, but that was OK because Mummy still did a lot and she was always there and he had time on his own with her.

There is nearly a four year gap between him and his younger brother and by this time things began to change. He was by now at school and, apart from Mummy disappearing for spells into hospital and having to grow up and be responsible quickly, he probably didn't notice it too much at first.

His younger brother on the other hand never had quite so much to do with Mummy as he grew. Daddy was the one he naturally turned to for help and as Daddy was at work for a lot of the time, he had to rely more and more on our helpers.

For several years it worked fine and then we began to notice it telling on both boys in little ways. They began to resent all the helpers and the constant stream of comings and goings of different people. It had its perks in some ways. They had lots of friends and occasional treats and people to take notice of them, but it wasn't really normal. You could tell that sometimes, coming home from school, they just wanted Mum or Dad and not always a visitor who was taking Mum's attention.

Mum too was deteriorating fast. The very things I had been able to cope with I had to let go of. Struggling with the house, family, driving and cooking was becoming too much and, because I was struggling, by the time my husband came home from work I was exhausted. Quite often we would wave the helper 'goodbye' and then Chris would help get me to bed, see to tea, put the boys to bed, and finally flop down in a chair to spend a lonely and fretful evening.

Life became one long joyless effort with little or no break. Even weekends weren't much fun with Chris having to catch up on chores - his and mine! All our church activities came to a halt. I was too ill to be involved and Chris was too busy looking after us all. The children could never really have friends round.... Mummy could never cope. Neither did we have friends around to entertain, and friends or relatives to stay became a thing of the past.

Our own relationship was obviously on the verge of suffering from such a strain. We were often like ships passing in the night: my husband coming home and me going to bed! He had to take more and more time off work to be with me and to see to the children because, although we had plenty of willing helpers, there were areas they could no longer really help with.

At first Chris was granted compassionate leave. Things improved for a while but this couldn't go on for ever. He was encouraged to work part-time with a view to gradually getting back to work completely. This too was OK until he tried returning to work full-time, and then we were back to square one. It was obvious a decision had to be made. Had he been able to take part-time work he might well have done so but this was not available. Anyway, he felt rather in limbo working part-time and spending the rest of the week at home catching up on chores and looking after the family. He was being torn between the two and could not give his full time and attention to either.

We did talk with our Christian friends and family and were even fortunate to know professional helpers who were Christians. Yet, amongst all these, nobody was able to support and advise us. It was certainly not through lack of concern but more through ignorance. They had been able to supply practical help, support, prayer and counsel in other areas but now they, like us, were out of their depth.

We did not realise until this point how very alone and isolated we were. Becoming a carer had never really been an issue for Chris to consider. He was married to me and he just stepped into the role. I could cope with help and, as we had plenty of volunteers, there was never any question about what his role should be. It just happened.

We needed advice about the way ahead and whether Chris should give up work, but there was none available. People only looked at the externals. The fact that my husband was still young and was being asked to give up his career so prematurely and be tied to a woman's world seemed to be the main concern. They felt he would be creating many problems, that he would feel resentful and unfulfilled and perhaps plain bored, and that it wouldn't work. They also saw no reason why the present practical arrangements could not continue and be expanded upon to allow him to stay at work.

What they all ignored completely, or perhaps just failed to understand, was our present existence. After all what is the point in saying 'I'm a man, my role is to go out to work and provide for my family, I have a career and ambition to fulfil' when one is being torn apart by circumstances and when life is just becoming a mere struggle for survival and existence. Perhaps when this happens it is time to stop and reassess and see just what God wants us to do.

I don't think anyone was able to see how it could possibly be in the will of God for Chris to give up work and how He could use us in this way. If I'm honest I don't think even we realised how God could bring something good out of it. But, eventually, we reached the point of seeing that the first move was with us and that we had to step out in faith towards what we believed was the right move and that good would follow. We had to be willing to change and adapt the roles we had been clinging to as our circumstances were changing fast. If we felt this way, how much more others must feel when they don't have the support of the one to be cared for or don't have a personal faith.

Becoming a carer may be difficult but it is never dull. It is like embarking on a voyage of discovery. Perhaps because my disease has been a gradual thing, in some ways, our voyage of discovery did not really begin until Chris needed to change the whole course of his life and give up work. For others the change may happen overnight. How or when it happens does not really matter.

The important thing, having established what one's caring role is to be, is to allow time for a period of general adjustment to the new role. However limited or difficult the relationship is between the carer and the person to be cared for, there will be a time to adjust to each other too. The lives of both are so tightly interwoven. There will be plenty of problems both mental and physical to cope with as one sets forth but before these are explored further perhaps it would be sensible to look at these periods of discovery in greater detail.

Chapter 4
A TIME OF DISCOVERY

Overnight and without warning Susan became a carer. Her husband suffered a severe stroke and the changes were enormous. One minute they were a normal, busy couple with a seven year-old daughter, running a country pub, the next minute the bottom had dropped out of their world.

The next few weeks passed in a kind of haze for Susan as she sought to run the business single-handed, look after her daughter and visit her husband in a hospital 40 miles away. She functioned automatically with little time to contemplate the future.

But their lives had changed for good. Her husband, Colin, always the strong 'front man', had altered beyond recognition. He had regained the use of his arms and legs to a certain extent and was able to feed and dress himself. However, his speech was limited and the words that had returned were liberally spiced with foul language ... something he'd always frowned upon. Worst of all he no longer saw Susan as his wife. 'Mammy' she became and 'Mammy' she remained for the three years which have followed. Somewhere inside he recognized that he needed her as a child needs a mother to care for him, to love him and to carry him.

Susan, always happy to stay in the background, recognized the new role that was to be hers and the changes that needed to be made. Six months after the stroke she gave up the business and they moved out. There would be other problems to face but she carried on without any thought for herself. She was functioning like a robot and, with hindsight, sees she was on the verge of going under. But eight months after the stroke, in spite of all the difficulties and the changed relationship, they had their 'moment of discovery' together.

The Hoover wouldn't work so Susan pulled it apart. It had become blocked with fluff. She poked and prodded and swore (even she had succumbed to swearing) but to no avail. Colin came into the room to discover her on hands and knees, peering into the nozzle and frantically switching it on and off. Suddenly, a ball of fluff and dust flew in her face. She didn't know whether to laugh or cry but one look at Colin's puzzled expression just broke something inside. They were in each other's arms laughing and crying for the first time.

It was not going to be easy, but from then on this was the start of the slow, upward struggle. Much of it would have to be without her husband's support but she began to look outside for that strength. She received help from others, and although she may not yet attach a 'God' label to it, she speaks of an inner strength and peace, and a feeling of not being alone. She is dealing with the feelings of resentment, bitterness and guilt that the whole situation has caused and is beginning to reach out and help others. She would probably be the first to admit she hasn't yet arrived and that there are plenty of day-to-day worries to deal with but from that one moment of discovery she has made a new beginning in accepting and learning to live with their situation.

We didn't have any one 'moment of discovery' like Susan and Colin. We had had plenty of things to deal with in the past and expected more in the future but, when Chris gave up work, we went through a kind of a honeymoon period which lasted a month or two. It was like being in the calm patch in the eye of a storm where all the most intense pressures were suspended for a time as we rediscovered ourselves and each other. It was an important time which gave us direction and stability for the way of life which was to follow.

From Day One of Chris leaving work we knew we had made the right choice. The sense of relief and peace was overwhelming and has remained. We spent a few weeks simply unwinding and enjoying it all before we began our new way of life in earnest. One of the first advantages we became aware of was that we started to operate as a family again. We began to relax and enjoy being on our own. It was good to see friends calling round for the children and being able to invite them in. Chris was able to concentrate on looking after us all and I was able to concentrate more time on the children ... chatting, helping with homework, reading and nurturing them spiritually, and they have obviously benefited greatly. Their Dad was also on hand to take and fetch them from school and do more active things with them like swimming and walking.

Our own relationship benefited. Instead of Chris only seeing me when I was flat out we were able to take advantage of my better state of health during the daytime. This meant outings and visiting people as well as just doing the chores together. Then, when I retired early, it didn't matter so much as we'd spent time together during the day. Another positive area was the fact that Chris was always on hand. There would be no more worries that the children were missing out on care, which should be at least one parent's responsibility.

Even better, it was such a relief to know Chris was not just there always to perform the essential daily tasks but that he was there on the bad days. The nature of my disease is such that I'm not just physically handicapped but also ill. Some periods are better than others but some dark spells last for months after which I never really fully pick up. All this is a strain on us both. It is just as hard to watch a loved one in a state of continual suffering as it is to be in it oneself. But at least we could now both be comforted by the fact that we were in the best situation we could be. When one is feeling really ill there is nothing more reassuring than to know that one can be put to bed and one's personal needs can be attended to by a loved one rather than a virtual stranger or in hospital or even by a friend. There is nothing better than the peace and quiet of one's own home to be oneself.

For Chris's part he no longer had to be away from home worrying or feeling guilty and then returning at night tired and yet still having to perform many jobs. That was real pressure! After the initial few weeks of unwinding there was a further period of discovery when we needed to work out quite a lot of practical implications and details and begin to adapt to our new roles. Each day we ventured on new ground.

For me, it meant learning to let go of the last remaining areas I was still struggling with and allowing Chris to take over. Slowly I passed on my 'expert advice' about how to clean and cook and shop and run the house. It took a lot of communicating and understanding and prayer. It was so easy for me to be critical and nagging and expect Chris to be some glorified robot functioning as my hands and feet and ready to obey every command my still very active brain was making. Frustrating for me but utterly soul-destroying for him!

For him, it was a whole new way of life. He had to accept advice and perform roles and functions totally alien to him and at the same time look after me more and more.

We came to realize that men and women are different and we must accept each other as we are. For instance, it was no good my sitting there and fuming at all the jobs which needed doing whilst my husband was able to relax over a cup of tea and well earned break. Just one lesson to be learned ... that some people keep going and others can switch off! There were countless other lessons on both sides but gradually a pattern and way of life emerged which now is very fulfilling.

Mary discovered that she and her husband had to learn similar lessons although the roles were reversed. She had no problems with her husband releasing the house to her. Quite the opposite! When he gets up his first thoughts go towards reading the newspaper regardless of the state the house is in! Her problem was with driving. Her husband became a back-seat driver and his cries of 'There's a sharp bend here' and 'Change down to third' drove her to distraction!

More recently we have been able to launch out more. Church activities have become possible again within our limitations. We can have the occasional visitors round and even people to stay because my husband is more than competent to deal with all the arrangements. We are learning what we are able to do and are building on this. People have to accept us as we are and, on this basis, it is surprising what a full life we have.

Shortly after our 'voyage of discovery' my specialist looked at me in a very concerned way and said: 'And what do you do with yourself all day?' obviously picturing a life of boredom. In the same way, our social worker looked at my husband kindly and said 'Have you really considered all the possibilities and help which are available to you and which would enable you to get back to your career before it is too late?' We were really taken aback and looked at her in utter amazement. We were so at peace and satisfied with our set-up it had never occurred to us that people still considered it not the ideal arrangement for us and as Christians, of course, we were quite content to accept the situation as being part of God's plan. It may not have been of our choosing but it was where He wanted us at that moment, and to strive and struggle after anything else would not make for happiness and our peace would vanish.

Perhaps that has been our most important discovery of all. Not just that God will remove all our problems like some glorious magician (although He can and does) but that He can be there with us in them. Knowing Him better and letting Him be part of our lives has given us a joy and peace which was never present before, even when our circumstances were normal. This has enabled us to carry on.

Each person's 'discovery time' is very personal. It may be a sudden incident or a gradual dawning. It may take a few months or a few years to happen. Problems will almost certainly appear before that. But I wanted to mention it first, before embarking on all the difficulties, because I feel it is very important to keep a positive view to the fore. It is very easy to start off negatively and remain so, and in trying to present a case paint a picture solely of doom and gloom. This is not honest or helpful. We have been down some pretty dark tunnels but always there has been light at the other end and, as Christians, we have always been aware of God giving us His love, joy, peace, strength, guidance and protection in the situations we have found ourselves.

Chapter 5
HELP!

'Asking for help is one of the hardest things so many of us find to do' says Susan. Help, whether advice or that of the practical kind, is certainly not always easy to come by. Neither is it easy to sort out what sort of help is required. But help is nearly always needed. In our case, different kinds of help were needed at different times. We were quite aware of the fact that we needed assistance from the moment I fell ill and even well before my condition had been officially diagnosed. But being willing to receive and accept help was quite another matter and was one of the first battles we had to face. It took several years to overcome and we could have saved ourselves a lot of hardship had we learned our lessons more quickly!

At first, it was all new and it seemed as if Chris could cope and that I would be able to manage reasonably well too. As a Christian it is easy to feel that one ought to be able to cope completely unaided (apart from God's help) and that to ask for assistance is a sign of failure! But God works through people and, although He does supply our every need, He often uses human agencies to do so.

It is good to recognize that we are only human so that when problems arise they need to be dealt with before they threaten to overwhelm and consume. Some are purely practical whereas others are far more deep rooted and personal and are to do with our minds, emotions and spirits. All can be dealt with but it needs not only carer and cared for (where possible) to be willing to admit they need help and to be open about it but also for people to be willing to listen and help.

People cannot help if they are unaware of the need and neither can they offer the best help if they do not fully understand the problem. It is up to the carer and their dependant to be willing to seek out the help which is available and, having discovered it, to be willing to actually ask for it. On the surface this seems a very obvious statement to make. Of course it might be, but I'm fully aware that knowing the right thing to do and actually stepping out to do it are two very different matters. This applies to many situations not just this one.

Some carers do not in fact want help even if this would be sensible. There are several reasons for this and it would be worthwhile to explore them in detail.

Through bitter experience we have discovered some answers and ways of overcoming these blockages to receiving help, and it would be good to share these too.

An Invasion of Privacy

People do not like an invasion of their privacy and would do anything to keep it, even to the point of struggling on unaided. Such a decision often means the situation becomes worse and worse. Fatigue and tiredness are closely followed by depression and in this state one becomes completely withdrawn and introverted. People become quick to criticize the lack of support, care and help and will even criticize that which is offered, and yet have no real intention of making use of anybody or anything. They become silent martyrs not caring saints and very little can be done for them!

I do understand because we've been there. We needed help right from the beginning. There was no question of struggling on unaided if Chris were to continue with his job. But we didn't want to accept the help, and in many ways didn't like it when it was given.

The invasion of privacy affected us both for 10 years. This was the period when I needed a lot of help especially in bringing up the children. I could manage in other areas and Chris didn't need to give up work, but because the children were of preschool age, I needed almost constant supervision.

This meant people were nearly always in our home during the working week. This affected me the most as Chris was at work all day. I used to treasure the weekends and occasional time to myself. The biggest treat for me was when people offered to take the children out or take them to their own houses for a few hours. I wouldn't have wanted this all the time. I wanted to share in the upbringing of them as much as possible, even if only as an onlooker. The treat was more about having a break from my helpers than my children! It really did me good and I was able to carry on again with renewed vigour.

But it affected Chris too, and one of the few things that really stands out in his memory was always returning home to finding someone else in the home. He seldom complained or said much, but I was aware that having had a busy day at work he would have preferred to have come in and just greeted his family or flopped in a chair for five minutes. Instead he always had to stand on ceremony and politely greet them. It was not that they stayed for ages after he had returned - they didn't - but rather the fact that they were there at all.

Knowing how he felt, I often politely tried to hint that they really didn't need to stay until he returned and that he'd soon be home. But they were so dutiful and loving that they never took the hint! It would have been far better to have been honest and told them straight and then we would have all known where we were, but we were too timid to do so.

Such a thing seems very small and silly now but at the time it seemed large and, as it went on for such a long period, it grew. These seemingly insignificant details are just the very thing which got on top of us and prevented us from wanting to receive help and they needed to be recognised and dealt with. If only we had done so we would have saved a lot of discomfort and misunderstanding.

People do things differently from us

Another problem area for us was the fact that people helped but they did things differently from us. They either took over and everything got done but not quite as we would have liked, or they expected us to tell them exactly what to do. When they lacked initiative we didn't like to put on them or appear too bossy so I usually ended up doing the task myself when they'd gone. Worse still, if it was a task I couldn't manage, poor Chris had to set to after a hard day's work!

It is so easy to imagine that we are indispensable and that nobody else can do things properly. This is just pride. Of course, there will be things that only the carer can manage or things which the dependant is not happy in letting anyone else do. This is fine, kept in perspective, and one can either work round these or accept them as inevitable. However, there are always some areas where one can let go and be helped. I can only say that through years of such experience we are learning to let go. What does it really matter if things are not quite done our way? If they are done and someone can take some of the strain off us, then we must be thankful and use the extra time that allows as is best for us.

We stand on ceremony

If one has accepted help it is best to move away and let the person get on with it. Easier said than done! The tendency is to watch over the helper either because one doesn't trust the person to do the job properly or because it seems impolite to leave them and go off and do your own thing. The helper will feel harassed and unable to perform the task properly, and usually the time is wasted anyway because you both spend the time talking and drinking cups of tea!

Chris has not actually had to face this problem yet because since leaving work he has always been fit and well, both physically and mentally, and has not needed to ask for this kind of help. When people call at inconvenient times he is quite happy to carry on with what he is doing, but this is probably because he knows I can entertain them. Although one can never be sure of how one will react in any given situation, I rather suspect he would be able to cope with helpers better than I did.

I spent years feeling I had to entertain my helpers and, as I had a regular procession of them, at the end of each day I felt quite worn out. I'm sure I made the invasion of privacy worse than it should have been by reacting in this way as I never felt I could relax and be myself. I always seemed to be waiting for someone to arrive and take over and never felt I could get on with something else while they were there. What a lot of wasted hours there must have been and how much more profitably could they have been spent! All the more so because many of my helpers actually asked me if I wanted to go and have a rest or something. Perhaps if I had done so I wouldn't have felt so worn out when my children and husband came home.

Guilt

We felt guilty. We felt we were putting on people even though they may have offered to help.

Mistrust

We felt that people didn't really want to help but had offered out of duty. Even if we accepted they wanted to help we felt they wouldn't want to keep it up and the situation would become awkward.

Most of our fears were totally unfounded and had we been more open we would have saved ourselves a lot of worry and anxiety. It is so easy to say this with hindsight but we should have been willing to trust people's words. Many people did genuinely want to help. People want to feel needed and useful, and some are just plain bored and looking for something to do. Many Christians would have offered in obedience to God's guidance. Whatever the motives, we should have been more willing to accept the help we have sometimes stifled or rejected. This was wrong when we did it for the wrong reasons.

Fear of and frustration at being let down

With government cut-backs some services for the disabled have been reduced or withdrawn. Dorothy is elderly and arthritic herself and yet cares for an 88 year old husband. 'My greatest frustration,' she says 'is that the various helps or visitors one may call upon for aid all "fizzle out" over a period of time due mainly to constant cut-backs. The home help is very good but severely limited as to hours.' Even with voluntary help people fear being let down. We were very blessed in the help we received but for some this is not always the case and such a situation would make people very reluctant to ask again.

So please, potential helpers, don't offer if you don't mean it or are not very reliable. It can do far more harm than good. Someone may have spent months plucking up courage to accept your help and if you let them down by starting off keen and then fading away, it will take a long time for them to trust someone else again. Carers have to be reliable and keep going however they feel and they will expect the same qualities from you.

Perhaps having help on a trial basis to begin with would be a sensible arrangement. In this way no one gets hurt and it gives both parties the option of withdrawing if it is obviously not working out.

Circumstances change

The carer may no longer need the help or the helper may no longer be able to give it and yet neither feel able to broach the subject. To avoid hurting each other, it would be far better to be open and honest enough to review the situation once in a while.

This was one area, at least, in which we personally had no trouble as many of our situations came to an end naturally. One helper married and moved away, another became pregnant and another took a full-time job. For our part some of the help naturally came to an end as the children grew older and more independent. In all these events we parted happily and we never felt let down or that we had hurt anyone either.

Suitability

Some help is not always suitable or adequate. This is particularly true of statutory help. But with voluntary help this can also be the case. People will sometimes offer help which they think we need. We were timid and did not like to seem unappreciative. But one should not feel pressurized into accepting help one doesn't feel is right or necessary. This will only have the effect of making one withdraw more for fear of feeling forced into unwanted situations and therefore miss out on the help that is needed.

It is sometimes hard to remember that one is still in charge of the situation and can accept as little or as much help as one wishes. Perhaps it is best to think small at first. An hour's help once a week can be a real lifesaver and give a much needed break. In the early days, because we felt awkward and didn't really want any help, we tended to let everyone do their own thing and consequently some of the help was not really wanted and some help that was needed was not given.

We have since discovered that it's much better to be honest. For instance, my husband can do almost everything now and has had a go at mending. However, it doesn't come naturally and neither has he the time to spend learning. When someone offered to do our ironing for us he said he didn't mind ironing and we don't do much anyway but could she do some mending instead? She didn't mind at all and the arrangement seems to work very well.

Inability to receive

'It is more blessed to give than receive' may be a true saying, but it is also certainly easier and you don't have to be a carer to find that out! Most of us like to give in whatever way we can and are often most willing to offer help where needed. It fulfils a need in us. Most people, if they're honest, would prefer not to be on the receiving end! It is fine for a short time. Have you ever been cossetted and pampered when you've been laid up with flu? Cups of tea, meals in bed, boxes of chocolates, flowers ... are all marvellous!

If the care extends to friends and neighbours rallying round and helping out that can be nice too. Offering to mind the children for an hour while you have a sleep or to do a bit of shopping or even the surprise meal left on the doorstep ... most of these are acceptable and welcome. Indeed they can be 'lifesavers', and one testifies afterwards to the wonderful support and care received and even to God's wonderful provision and timing in supplying help just when it was most needed. It is made even more acceptable by the thought in the back of your mind telling you 'When I'm better, I'll be able to do something in return.'

All this is the normal way of things and is common to most people's experience. Wonderful and fine and thank goodness for it, but have you ever been thrown into the situation where you know you're going to need help for a long time? It's not so easy to ask for and accept it then! We like our independence and we don't want to be beholden to anyone. We feel so useless and such a nuisance. Also, it's OK to receive when you know you'll be able to return the favour sometime but what if you know you can't? To receive, receive and receive again is really hard.

We really had no choice but to accept because we were desperate and people were wonderful to us. But if I'm honest it was a really hard thing to do week after week, month after month, year after year. I used to long to do something back and fret because we couldn't. I concentrated on the things I couldn't manage, like offering to mind other people's children for them or entertaining. I also felt guilty because I was stopping Chris from doing these things too ... by my very existence!

I failed to see the areas (small though they were) where we could give back and anyway at that stage would have been doing so for the wrong reasons. It would not have been so much out of love or where a need arose which we could fulfil but more to repay a debt or return a favour.

I'm sure this state of affairs is not just common to dependants or carers but to lots of others too. Single parents, the elderly and the poor spring to mind. The phrase 'I'm not accepting charity' is a well worn one. But how silly and proud! There is a real blessing to be had in receiving just as in giving. It has to be a reciprocal arrangement though. There are of course the 'takers' in society who drain and sponge and put people out but they are only a small minority. It is far more common to find those who are so willing to give but so unable to receive.

Gradually, however, I discovered that as I received, God changed me and receiving was no longer a problem. I began to be able to accept things without even wanting to repay. I began to see the love behind the actions and see Jesus' love itself being made manifest through ordinary people. What right had I to spurn such love and also to spoil the kindly act and hurt the person offering it?

It was when I was able to accept quite big things which I knew were quite sacrificial on the part of the giver, that I knew I was being changed. For instance, there was the beautiful shawl knitted for me to keep me warm. It must have been quite time consuming and costly and it was given by someone with little spare time or money. How awful if I'd spoiled it all by saying 'You shouldn't have, I can't possibly accept that.'

If God was altering my attitudes He was doing the same work in Chris too because many acts of receiving involved us both. On one occasion we kept receiving beautiful boxes of fruit and vegetables on our doorstep after I'd been particularly ill. After two or three deliveries with more food than we could manage, we thought we'd better find out who was responsible. We feared the greengrocer may have got the message wrong, that the person had only intended a single box of groceries and would be shocked by a big bill.

In finding out who was sending the goods we probably spoiled it a bit as the person had wished to remain anonymous, but what they said was lovely. They felt so concerned because they couldn't do anything to make me better so they had done the only thing they could and expressed their love in a practical way.

I'm sure they are no better off than we are and we didn't 'need' it as such. Two good reasons to refuse. Yet we accepted with the proviso that they must not feel obliged to carry on for ever, but only for as long as they felt led to and we also halved the quantity, as we just couldn't get through it all! I didn't really expect it to be quite the blessing it is. We don't need it but the joy of getting a surprise box of goodies every week and understanding the depth of love behind it is tremendous. During hard times it has really lifted us. Just to know of that constant and faithful love week by week has really reminded us of God's faithfulness and constancy.

Having been brave enough to step out and start receiving, it has now really become quite easy to do and I really feel that we have learned an important lesson and have overcome what was once a problem. In so doing we have such a sense of release. We no longer feel bound to give in return or pay back but just accept willingly what people offer. Gone is the need to only give Christmas cards and presents to those who give to us and to get in a stew about an unexpected card or present which arrives late. We give where we want and expect nothing in return. Gone is the need to offer payment for every stamp or telephone call if it is quite obvious the person doesn't want it. Neither do we expect to return every cake or bunch of flowers which come our way.

It wasn't until we began to receive willingly that God showed me something else, an added bonus. This was quite simply the realization that we were able to give too! We were no longer giving to repay a favour, and indeed the people we were able to give to were not necessarily the ones who had given to us.

After my husband became a full-time carer, we discovered all sorts of ways of being 'useful' without even trying. A whole new world opened up. In his 'spare' time he gives a lot to others, whether it is running errands for my elderly parents whilst doing our shopping, or doing the odd job for somebody, or even doing a bit of extra baking. He is extremely busy and tied by me but it is amazing how you can always manage to do something for someone if you want to. It is just a question of accepting one's limitations and operating within them.

Some may think their limitations are so severe that they can give nothing. Well, we have times when this is how it feels for us too but there is always something we have to offer, however small it may seem to us, and often we are quite unaware of giving it. I used to feel sorry for those that had to look after us so much, imagining it was done out of duty rather than anything else. But every now and again people say something encouraging (probably without realizing it) and, when I've pieced all the snippets together I actually begin to believe we have something to offer just by 'being' and not by doing anything at all.

People say ours is a peaceful house and that they like coming round even if it is to sit for the children and me because they enjoy the break and a chance to chat and relax. Someone called the other day on an errand and stayed about an hour. I didn't feel as if we'd done anything for them ... indeed I think we did most of the talking! But before leaving they said how much they had enjoyed the time spent with us (they spend so much time in helping and counselling people with so many problems) and that it had made such a welcome break from trying to sort people out. I had been feeling guilty at taking up their time and feeling the gain was all on our side, so I was amazed.

Just recently, a friend of my mother-in-law, who we had never even met, made me a muff. Mum-in-law had mentioned to her that I would like to have a muff to keep my hands warm as gloves are not very easy to manage. She was asking her if she knew how she could make one for me. Without saying anything to my Mum, this kind lady spent ages shopping for some suitable fabric, designing and then making a muff for me. It would have been so easy to tell her off and refuse to accept it without paying for it, but instead we gratefully received it and arranged to meet her at my Mum's for a meal to say 'thank you' and to introduce ourselves. Before this meeting took place, we were out shopping one day and I was seated in my wheelchair, wearing my muff. Somebody stopped us saying 'I know who you are. You must be Brenda. I recognize my muff.' When we eventually met properly, she confided that it had made her day seeing me out and wearing it. Just by 'being' we had given her as much pleasure as she had given us!

So if you can't 'do' just 'be'. There are lots of doers about anyway and people may prefer a 'be-er' for a change! If you're a helper rather than a carer or dependant, don't forget that you can offer such words of encouragement too which will do so much to restore a sense of worth and value to life and help carers and dependants to realize they are not doing all the taking.

As already stated it is not always right to accept help. It may not be suitable or what we have in mind at all and we need to consider every offer carefully, especially if it will be help given on a regular basis.

As Christians, there were some marvellous occasions when God showed us in very special ways that, despite the difficult circumstances,

He was in complete control and cared and that He wanted us to trust Him. We needed to learn that, first and foremost, having committed our lives to God, we should learn to depend on Him for our needs. These were the times when we needed help, usually because our normal helpers were unable to come, but felt it wrong to make any alternative arrangements, believing God would supply our needs. And He always did.

Some of our helpers would get in quite a flap, feeling they had let us down, and offering to arrange all sorts of elaborate alternatives. At such times there would be an enormous sense of peace and we would politely refuse their frantic efforts saying 'It's Okay, don't worry, it'll all work out, just leave it.'

One week of such occasions stands out in my mind. I was very ill and confined upstairs as I could no longer manage the stairs. Up until then we had managed very well mainly with the help of our relatives. But my condition was putting increasing demands on them and they were getting tired and unable to cope. We really didn't know what to do and were very loth to accept outside help, but it was as if God was showing us how much He cared and that we were to trust Him over the whole matter.

On Sunday a friend arrived with some baking ... and Chris had been struggling all day to get round to doing some.

On Tuesday I told my Mum-in-law that two friends had offered to help in any way and asked whether she would like me to phone them to see if they would be able to give her a break for a morning. She suggested Thursday so that she could go shopping. I was a bit doubtful that they would be able to manage Thursday but said I'd ask. Before I could do so the telephone rang. It was them, of course, offering help for the whole of Thursday! Not only did she get her morning shopping trip but my parents were able to have the afternoon off too.

On Wednesday there was no help available to us for the first part of the afternoon. Chris returned home for lunch and then I was alone. I was pretty helpless. Being left with two small children was bad enough but, on this particular occasion, the elder child was supposed to be going to a party, and there was no way to get him there. But before Chris returned to work our need had been met. My father called in unexpectedly and offered to take him. I was not too happy about this as my father is very elderly and also rather lame and I didn't feel he would be able to cope with a lively four year-old. But at least there was someone to keep an eye on me and the toddler. In the end everything was fine because just before the time of the party a friend called and was only too willing to take him.

However, such occurrences were not the norm and not the way God expected us to carry on. We needed to accept more help from 'outsiders' and plan carefully.

This was a hard step to take. Only an extended stay in hospital and major surgery forced us to admit defeat. At this point, someone virtually took the situation out of our hands by supplying us with many willing helpers and convincing us that we ought to let them all help. Some help we did have to refuse but only because it wasn't suitable or easy to implement.

Some people may still feel unable to ask for help on these terms. But there is probably professional or paid-for help which can be considered as an alternative. Indeed, we supplemented our help with help from the social services, partly because we didn't want to impose on anyone else and partly because it was nice to have some help from people who were not related or linked to us by ties of friendship.

It doesn't really matter which kind of help it is. Different kinds will be more suited to different people or circumstances. The main thing is to be willing to seek help when it is required.

Once we gave up the struggle it all worked out really well and we saw the folly of not accepting help sooner. Over the years our helpers became our constant friends and companions and we really grew to love them. Even now, after several years without their help, some remain very special to us both because of the things we went through together. It was not all a one way thing. I know they feel the same and also have a soft spot for the children, having had so much to do with them in their early years. By accepting their help, even though we didn't want it, we have not only been enabled to cope but have also gained and learned so much from the experience.

Perhaps it is now time to explore, in greater detail, some of the problem areas. It would be impossible to explore them all in one chapter! The practical issues requiring help are often linked to one's emotional and spiritual needs. It is very hard to separate them. Sometimes we can help ourselves, sometimes others can help us, but if we are to become really whole we will need to accept help from God too.

Chapter 6
LOVE: AN IMPOSSIBILITY OR THE KEY?

'I loved my parents - as they were originally - but they became different people as their illness progressed,' says Gladys, whose parents both suffered from arteriosclerosis which caused severe mental problems. One morning she counted thirteen cups of tea in her bedroom! Her Father, a sweet-natured person, had always brought her a cup of tea in bed and woken her as she had to leave the house early for work. As his mind deteriorated, night and day merged, and throughout the night he would bring her cups of tea and tell her to get up. There are countless similar episodes she could recount. As an only child and also unmarried, she spent years caring for her parents alone and feeling very isolated.

Sadly, Gladys describes the whole experience as 'hell' and, when her parents eventually died, the only way she was able to come to terms with the whole 'nightmare period' was to move to the other end of the country and make a new life for herself. A doctor said 'This has marred you for life. You will never get over it.' A foolish thing to say, she thought, but she has since discovered that this has indeed been the case, in spite of trying to make a new start elsewhere.

There must be times in many people's lives when love seems an impossibility. For a carer, in a difficult situation like Gladys, there is quite a strong possibility that this will be the case. Does it have to be as despairing and tragic as Gladys' experience or is there any hope that such severe problems can be overcome?

One of the most well known and loved passages in the Bible defines what love is: it is patient, kind and unselfish. It is not irritable or resentful. It bears, believes, hopes and endures all things (1 Corinthians 13). All very well, but what an impossibility!

How can one love someone anymore when they have changed out of all recognition, either mentally or physically? How does one love someone who is totally confused or going senile or experiencing wild swings of mood or personality? How can one communicate with them anymore? Love can quickly fade or become simply one's duty because the person is remembered as they once were and for all they have done in the past and therefore they are owed something.

As love diminishes, gratitude or duty, on their own, are not sufficient. If one performs one's tasks solely from these motives, there will be many failures or feelings of failure and guilt may well develop too. But if love has gone and such motives are inadequate how can one cope?

How can one love the person suddenly maimed or gradually deformed by disease? How can one deal with the feelings of revulsion that may arise? How can one love the handicapped baby when one spent nine months anticipating something quite different? How can one love the handicapped child who people stare at and whisper about? Impossible, or at least a big strain. Or is it? Can love be strengthened or restored?

God is Love

God is love and love comes from God (we are told in 1 John 4:7,8). This passage of scripture goes on to show that God made His love manifest to us by sending His son Jesus into the world to die for our sins. If we are honest with ourselves it is obvious that we all fall short of God's standards in so many ways. That's why the passage telling us how to love seems such an impossibility to live up to. By our own strength alone it is, and we will fail time and time again and get depressed about it. The more we long to live up to God's standards and the more a carer struggles to be loving when placed in some very difficult situations the more the person will fail. For we are not God and we are not perfect.

God loves me!

But God loves us and doesn't want us to struggle. He has offered us a way out in the form of Jesus Christ , His only Son. Jesus paid the price for all our failures by giving His life for us. This was necessary because God who is perfect and holy cannot look upon our failures and wrongs (the Bible calls this 'sin'). He requires a sacrifice to put things right. Jesus became this sacrifice for us. What love - to actually die for us!

We can be restored by love
and have a relationship with God

The good news is that if we accept this love for ourselves not only are we forgiven by God and our relationship with Him is restored - this brings great peace of mind in itself - but now God Himself will be able to come and dwell in us through Jesus' sacrifice. It was not possible before because we were separated and cut off from Him by all our failures (and failing to love is only one such area).

How?

How do we accept Jesus' sacrifice? Simply by giving up the struggle of trying to be good and admitting that we can't manage it. We can then acknowledge and accept that Jesus has done it all for us anyway and we needn't try anymore. He is the missing ingredient in our lives and if we are to get on top of this situation (and all other ones too) we must admit our need and ask God to come and take over from now on.

This is not an easy thing to do. We are not sure what it will mean and we like to control our own lives even when we see we are making a mess of things. Unfortunately, it is not until we step out in faith and hand ourselves over that we can really see the truth of this. We just have to trust Him over it and trust that what the Bible says is true. We have to be like Peter when he walked on water. It wasn't until he actually stepped out of the boat that he really knew for sure that he could walk on water.

God will live within us

Having taken the plunge, we suddenly discover it is true because God sends His own Spirit to come and live within us. His Holy Spirit starts to make things clear to us. It is not just a matter of facts anymore but the real God living within us, making us aware of His presence and making it possible for us to live as He wants us to.

How will all this make us more loving?

As one of God's characteristics is love, gradually, as we allow Him to, He will pour His love into us and it will be perfected in us. One of the 'fruits' (or evidences) of the Holy Spirit dwelling inside us is love. We may not be aware of it at first but our attitudes will change and we will begin to become more like Jesus and more able to demonstrate the love shown in 1 Corinthians 13.

This may still seem impossible but after all if God died for us and offered us His love while we were unlovely and still in sin (Romans 5:7,8), is it not possible that He can give us love for the unlovely and for the unlovely situations in life?

We must keep our eyes on God though

All this can be true as long as we keep our eyes fixed on the source of that love and not on ourselves. As long as Peter had his eyes firmly fixed on

Jesus, he could walk on the water. As soon as he looked at himself again he started sinking.

Triumphant ... even if we fail sometimes

We can experience victory in this area however hard or slow our progress appears to us. The good thing is that we may fail but 'Love never ends' (1 Corinthians 13:8) and God is always there to forgive us and to pick up the pieces as we start again.

What of those who do not profess this faith and trust in the Lord Jesus Christ? Some of them are wonderful carers and indeed put some Christians to shame. How can they demonstrate the love they do and if they can manage it, why do we need God's help? The answer, I believe, is that we are all made by God and in His image. Love is one of His attributes and therefore we all display love to a greater or lesser degree. We still reflect the image of our Maker however marred and unclear that reflection has become through our own rejection and turning away from Him.

Some people are naturally more loving than others and can endure much and overcome much. Whether by nature or because of the environment we've been brought up in we all respond in different ways. However, if one is coping under one's own steam, it is much more of a strain. The pressure mounts and it is easy to crack and go under. How much better to be able to rely on the abundant supply of God's love, which He offers so freely, than to struggle with our own natural but weak and imperfect supply.

Christians of course are not exempt from pressures either but at least we have somewhere to take our problems. As we release them to God, He is able to step in and enable us to cope in His strength, and provide help and support through others too. However bleak and unlovely the situation He can give us His love.

This has been our experience. As I become more and more physically handicapped and deformed and as I see very few parts of my body unaffected in some way, it is very easy to look at the outward things and doubt how my husband could possibly still love me. How can he love me when he has to perform all the most intimate things which I would normally do for myself? My dignity and privacy have gone. I can no longer make myself look my best for him as he has to wash and dress me and comb my hair and clean my nails, and do a thousand and one even more personal things beside.

When I read some of the 'problem pages' and see what things are a real worry and problem to people - the most minute blemish becomes such a major catastrophe and people fear they will never be attractive to anyone

- then I realise what a work of grace and love God has been performing in our lives. The amazing thing is that we still love each other.

I realize that Chris does not have some of the problems that some carers have to cope with in that while I may not physically be the 'old me', my mind has not been affected and we can have a good relationship on that level. He has said to me 'well, you're still the same person inside and we can still be best friends and although our fun is limited, we can still have fun together.' I feel this must be an easier relationship to maintain than the one Gladys was faced with, i.e. with someone who can physically care for themselves and who looks normal but whose mind is affected. And I realize there are still others who care for someone sick in body and in mind.

However, there are some practical and spiritual tips which we and others have found helpful and which may be useful to consider.

Communication

It is important to try to share your feelings with your partner, however impossible this may appear. If speech is difficult try to keep in touch in other ways concentrating on what is possible now rather than what you have lost: touching, hugging, holding hands, listening to music, watching television, laughing, crying, praying together. All are simple and effective ways of maintaining a relationship . Susan, whose husband was affected by a stroke was able, as has already been mentioned, to keep the channels open by touching and hugging.

Carol had a good relationship with her mother who, when her sight deteriorated, came to live with her and her husband. Her mother was easy to get on with and seldom complained which must have made life easier but at the same time she recognizes that there were times when they became frustrated with each other. 'Guess we got a little tired of each other's faces!' But they used to spend time in the afternoons chatting together. Her mother would love to recall stories from her youth and she would love to listen. The relationship was strengthened by being able to talk and share together and twelve years after her mother's death, Carol still misses her.

When I was very ill and could do very little except be in bed and rest or sleep we discovered a shared joy in watching the birds together. Chris would collect scraps and even make bird food and hang them on the tree outside my window, and we spent many a happy moment watching their antics during the dark winter days.

Retain a degree of independence

Try to have some sort of independence and time away from each other so that you will come back to each other renewed and refreshed. It may be hard to arrange, and I'll deal with this more fully elsewhere, but even an hour's break once a week works wonders and most of us can probably manage more than this. As Mary put it, 'It's lovely to have the house to myself sometimes. It is knowing you have the freedom to do what you want when you want that's important.'

Dealing with feelings of revulsion

If a relationship causes feelings of revulsion, don't feel guilty. Instead be positive and think of ways around it. One idea is for carer and dependant to look upon dealing with such things as personal hygiene as purely a job to be performed. Look at yourselves as patient and nurse rather than husband and wife or mother and daughter etc. If the carer has a status in society and feels worth something this will help as he will feel he is performing his job of work and may find it easier to separate the personal involvement from the professional role he is maintaining.

If the feeling of revulsion remains, another way around it is to seek help from outside. Have a word with your G.P. or social worker. There are professional people who can take over some of these more personal aspects for you. District nurses can deal with medical problems and provide practical help with things like changing dressings, toileting and bathing etc. If a relationship is suffering because of such feelings or because the dependant himself would prefer to keep a degree of privacy, at times, it is also worth considering that care attendants can be provided through the health authority, social services and sometimes voluntary organisations. Such people are able to help with washing and dressing a person and as such can provide a valuable service.

None of these areas have greatly bothered us so far, as my husband is happy to do anything for me and I prefer it to be him doing it. However, in one small way I can understand the problem. The only thing Chris really hates the thought of is having anything to do with my teeth. The dentist has been urging him to help me clean them but so far we have resisted and I prefer to struggle on alone, not just because I know it revolts him but also because my gums and teeth get very sore and I prefer my gentle touch! However, we do appreciate that if the time comes we will have to get over the problem and it is vital to know we can share our feelings with each other about such things.

Sexual problems

Another area where things can go wrong is the whole question of sexual relationships between husband and wife. As well as the feelings of revulsion and no longer being attracted to one's partner there are other considerations.

We have been faced with the fact that it is no longer possible to make love in the way we used to or the way we would necessarily like. There have been times when just getting through each day may have been utterly exhausting, leaving no room for anything else.

So often, by the evening, I am feeling so ill and in so much pain that lovemaking is far from my mind and if my husband had had any romantic notions throughout the day they have to be well and truly repressed. Indeed, he doesn't wish to cause me any more pain and so it is easy for him to repress such feelings altogether.

For my part I have suffered severe feelings of guilt that I cannot be the wife I should be to him and have felt it would be better if I were to die and release him. It has been vital for us to keep the channels open in our marriage and share these things. There are ways around some of these problems if we are only willing to admit and face them together, and even if some problems are insurmountable at least sharing them together has brought us closer whereas we may have drifted apart, isolated by our own private sorrow.

Personally, I have found that when I brought the whole area to God things changed too. For years it was an area I kept Him out of. One doesn't talk about such things, especially to God! But I discovered that He cared about this as much as any other area of our lives. The problems haven't all been removed but I find our relationship is far sweeter and deeper than it was and although limited in some senses also totally satisfying. God has made it so as we have allowed Him to.

Some types of mental illness can cause odd sexual behaviour and may be very distressing to the carer. It may not be possible to share with one's partner if they are mentally disturbed or perhaps just unwilling to do so. This must be really distressing and is certainly outside our experience. The only comfort I can offer is that God does understand and when we take such things to Him, He is able to help us.

Whatever the sexual problem and whether it must be tackled alone or with one's partner, there is professional advice to be sought. Relate (formerly the National Marriage Guidance Council) has local branches who can offer counsel. There is also an organisation called SPOD ... Sexual and Personal Relationships of People with a Disability (see chapter 13 on 'Where to get Voluntary Help' for the address) which provides information and service to clients and professionals.

Service

It is good to remember that one of the roles of the Christian is to serve others. (Mark 10:42-44). We are all called upon to do this but obviously some are called to a greater degree than others and a carer is one such example.

Jesus goes on to show that He is not asking us to do more than was required of Himself: 'For the Son of Man also came not to be served but to serve, and give His life to be ransomed for many' (Mark 10:45). In John's gospel (chapter 13:12-17) He speaks further about serving one another and indeed by His own action of washing the disciple's feet, sets the example and attitude to follow. So however menial or revolting the task, Jesus has been there first and if we give the situation over to Him, He will enable us to triumph over it and will bless us in it.

Trials and tribulations

For the Christian, it is also worth holding on to the thought that Jesus never promised us a bed of roses and a life of ease. Sometimes He calls us to be willing to suffer for Him and be willing to share in His suffering and the suffering of others. By doing this He not only refines us and makes us into the people He wants us to be but He also enables us to feel more compassion and love and care for a very needy world.

Linda discovered this truth. She had always had a difficult relationship with her mother who had had a very hard life and who resented her even being born. She had cared for Linda but had never really been able to show love or affection and was unable to accept help or love from Linda. This had resulted in Linda feeling inferior and of little value. So, when Linda's father, with whom she had a very good relationship, died first, she was very resentful as she would have much preferred looking after him. But her mother needed help and she did her best, despite many rebuffs and rejections, to offer it. It was not easy but she held on to the fact that God requires us not only to suffer sometimes but to take part willingly in our suffering! The Bible says 'Count it all joy when you meet various trials' (James 1:2). Such a thing would have been impossible with her own strength alone but as she learned to give the situation over to Him she was able to receive His love and help and to remain positive.

She persevered and gradually saw a change in her mother. She became more frail but also more appreciative and loving. Over the years a relationship was slowly built and they became much closer. Before her mother died she made a new will which made Linda the sole executor - a compliment indeed, showing that at last she was prepared to trust her fully with her affairs! Had Linda given up years before their relationship would never have been restored and Linda might still be struggling with feelings of guilt and resentment. As it is, she grieves and misses her mother in a completely natural way.

It is wonderful to know that God's love inside us will enable us to cope in all these situations whether our relationship is that of parent and child, husband and wife or friend to friend. Also, not only does He provide us with His love deep within but manifests it in many ways, often providing help and comfort through others too.

Chapter 7
SADNESS INTO GLADNESS

Each evening, on his way home from work, John used to call in to see his mother. One night, he nearly shot out of his chair as he heard the unexpected words: 'Who's the oldest, me or you?' With a sinking feeling he realized she was showing the first signs of senility.

We often associate the feelings of grief and loss with the actual death of a loved one. Some carers will be faced with the death of the one cared for, whether through age or illness or both. Some have been preparing themselves for the inevitable for months or even years and yet when it happens there are a mixture of feelings to contend with. There will be sadness, but it may be tinged with relief and guilt. I shall look at the carer who has been bereaved and some of the feelings they have to come to terms with in a later chapter.

But there are other kinds of bereavement which do not actually relate to dying.

* Grief comes from seeing a loved one changed from the person they once were. Illness, accident or age makes them a different person.

* Grief comes through dashed hopes and dreams of what might have been. It comes through the disappointment of knowing that the child you have borne is abnormal in some way. All the expectations and plans you had for them must be relinquished.

* Grief comes when you recognize that all these situations will affect you too. You will experience a loss of freedom. There will be opportunities and ambitions which will never be realised.

When confronted with such things there are three important points to remember and which we will investigate further. The first concerns the grieving process:

Take time to grieve

Grief should not be hurried. One of the books of wisdom in the Bible says there is a season and time for everything. There is a time to weep and a time to laugh; a time to mourn and a time to dance. (Ecclesiastes 3:4,5) Jesus himself wept when He heard of the death of His friend Lazarus. It is right and proper to show grief when a loss has been suffered.

Grief should not be stifled

Don't bottle up your feelings. The problem is that many people do not grieve. They stifle their emotions. They cope marvellously and present the 'stiff upper lip' at all times. They immerse themselves in activity from dawn 'til dusk and often end up with far more problems to work through and even complete breakdown.

Don't be afraid to take time to be alone with yourself and perhaps with God. There is a time for examining and coming to terms with your feelings. You may respond in anger or weeping or by becoming quiet and withdrawn. You may prefer to work through it on your own or you may need to talk to someone.

If you want to talk to someone then be prepared to share with a friend or member of your family. Sometimes it is helpful to get in touch with a group who are involved with coping or caring for the same disability or illness as you are and who will understand the feelings of loss you are experiencing. There are more and more carer's support groups being set up too and these can be a good place to vent your feelings. (See chapter 13 on voluntary help). Be assured that whatever your loss such reactions are normal and natural and time needs to be given to them.

Both Chris and I have spent a long time over the years grieving and coming to terms with our losses. Some things such as loss of health and ability to do things you once took for granted are obvious. But there are many smaller areas which keep cropping up or which only become obvious in certain situations and which need to be dealt with too. But whichever situation we have found ourselves in, we have discovered the importance of grieving.

Personally, we have found that we have coped with the larger areas of loss more easily than the smaller things which have often taken us by surprise and threatened to upset and depress. For instance, we have learned how to be very fulfilled within our own home and set-up, and within our limitations we can cope and manage all sorts of things. When removed from these surroundings we can flounder.

We no longer attend big Christian gatherings, mainly it's true, because we are becoming more limited in our activities. However, another important factor is the sense of loss we experience. It is suddenly brought home to us that we cannot do as every one else does and so often we have come home feeling frustrated, disappointed and upset. We are confronted with meetings we are not able to attend, activities we can't join in with and places we can't get to. It affects carer and dependant alike. But, in one way, perhaps it affects the carer even more because they, at least, would still be able to do such things were they free.

Even smaller gatherings become something to be avoided unless we organise them or know the situation we're invited to very well! I recall a picnic/walk which we felt we could join in with. My husband really needed a break of this kind as I was just recovering from a very bad spell. It took a lot of effort and planning to get there. We arrived a bit late and then saw the picnic site wasn't very suitable. It was nowhere near a loo and also involved crossing over a stream. We headed straight to the nearest town for a toilet and then got back in time for me to be carried over the stream in the wheelchair. We sat down as everyone was finishing their picnic and preparing to go on various walks. This we were prepared for, but we had expected a few people to remain, especially when they saw we were there. However, as so often happens, we became a dumping ground for goods and children and spent an exhausting couple of hours minding both. We couldn't go home even though I'd more than had enough, because of the children left in our charge and also because we couldn't get back over the stream without help! Thank God I didn't need the loo again!

Of course, one can't expect people to understand our every need but this sort of thing happens fairly frequently. People are wonderful in small groups or as individuals but a bit thoughtless when together. So we have learned to avoid people *en masse* and make our own pleasures and activities as suit us best.

This does not mean that we run and hide from our responsibilities. There are many situations we face where it would be far less painful to avoid them. Activities and functions for the children come to mind. We hate attending parents' evenings or coffee mornings where I am rammed into a corner and my husband tries to manoeuvre the wheelchair round tight spaces and lots of people holding coffee cups! It becomes a nightmare and an occasion of endurance rather than enjoyment.

I recall taking our elder son to his adventure holiday in the Peak District. It was a lovely place, with friendly staff to welcome us and in order to make the children feel at home before the parents departed, we were invited to stay for coffee. However, the dining room of a youth hostel filled to capacity with children, parents, rucksacks, walking boots and suitcases is not the ideal place to try and negotiate a wheelchair! We had already had a long journey and were well aware of the impending return trip but we would not have declined the invitation for anything. What was our sense of frustration, awareness of loss and inability to be part of the situation compared with seeing our son happy and settled?

Chris, in particular, has had to mourn the loss of many things. He has, of course, had to come to terms with the loss of his career fairly recently, but even before he gave up work, he had to cope with the fact that any ambitions job-wise could never be realized. His firm were very kind and understanding but he could never work overtime or go on courses to further his career.

His leisure activities have been curtailed too. He has always had a passion for steam and spent many a happy hour watching, listening to and photographing steam trains. Sometimes he used to go on special excursions. He was brought up by the sea and has always been used to swimming and boating. A holiday by the sea is no longer really suitable as access to beaches is very limited. I know he yearns to go off and have a go at surfing or some other popular water sport and this is now just not possible.

We live in the Lakes and have a dinghy from times past but it seldom gets used. He also would love to go stock car racing or watch wrestling or go to country and western concerts.

Experiences similar to these are sustained, to a greater or lesser degree by most carers. Len lost his job because he now cares for his physically disabled wife. He had to give up some hobbies too - not least, playing in a band every weekend. Helen and her husband have a mentally handicapped daughter. They also have a perfectly normal daughter and have had to accept that many normal family outings and activities are either not possible or fraught with difficulties.

The second important point to remember is that grieving is not supposed to last forever.

Time heals and God heals.

As we have been prepared to commit our grief to God we have seen that He can and does restore in His own time. The initial grieving period has played a vital part in the healing process but there comes a time to move on. We can be restored.

Many people do grieve but fail to see when the time of mourning is over. They concentrate on the loss and grief, becoming more and more introspective and negative and wallow in self pity. It's so easy to develop a negative attitude. But there are several areas in which we can help ourselves.

Cherish happy times both past and present

We remember with pleasure our first two years of marriage when things were normal: setting up our first home together, taking a holiday abroad, being involved in many activities and going out to work. We also store up happy times now: holidays, precious moments as the children grow up, outings, special treats, evenings when I am able to stay up a bit later and even manage to go out. All are treasured memories which help us through the bad times and which make us aware of God's goodness in so many little ways. Indeed, perhaps we no longer take things for granted and appreciate them all the more.

Helen finds shopping with her mentally handicapped daughter a bit of a nightmare and often buys items she doesn't want because her daughter has put them in her trolley. But recently shopping afforded a rare and unexpected pleasure. Her daughter stood in front of a market stall admiring the soft toys. They stayed there for some time and then Helen said that maybe Father Christmas would bring her one. The stall holder, on impulse, just reached over and gave her a beautiful soft toy cat. This was a moment to treasure!

Be positive

All the losses I have been describing have their positive side too. We need to concentrate on the things that are still available to us.

For instance, my husband may have lost his career prospects and no longer be able to go out to work but there are plenty of opportunities in his new way of life. He is available, during the daytime, to meet many needs. He can associate with other men who are perhaps unemployed, retired or working shifts. He has helped out in the children's primary schools and has been most welcome. Not many infant children have much contact with male teachers! He is able to do odd jobs for elderly people or single mums. It is a time for looking forward, not back.

With regard to leisure pursuits, Chris is learning to adapt them. He now turns his attention to model railways. We have a large attic upstairs and he can model and play up there to his heart's content (time permitting) and still keep an eye on me. Swimming and surfing in the sea may be out, but we have the Lake District on our doorstep with rivers and streams and lakes to mess about in. Len, who had to give up playing in the band, concentrates on writing and drawing cartoons.

Some things become an occasional treat rather than a frequent activity and are no less enjoyable for that. Helen and her family take an occasional weekend break or holiday without their handicapped daughter so that they can indulge in normal family activities, like swimming, which would otherwise be impossible.

Keep things in perspective

There is a temptation to behave like the children who are always saying 'Why can't I? Everyone else does!' We have usually discovered that there are lots of other reasons why 'everyone else' doesn't and that we only concentrate on the few who seem to have it all their own way. It's not only carers who experience such losses anyway. Poverty, one parent families, exacting jobs, bereavement and marriage failure all take their toll too and it's good to keep things in perspective.

Retain a sense of humour

'It's often easier to look back and laugh rather than cry' says Helen. I have talked to and received letters and stories from a variety of carers and for those who manage to cope and come to terms with things, this sentiment is expressed over and over again as an important remedy.

Where both carer and dependant are able to retain a sense of humour is obviously the best situation to be in. Like Anne whose her carer husband keeps her and the rest of the family in fits of laughter with his quick wit, usually at her expense. Sitting in the garden one day with him Anne said 'Will you move the umbrella', quickly followed by 'Put my glasses on the table love'. She then spotted a black cloud and remarked on it. Her husband quickly replied 'What would you like me to do with that?'

His antics amuse her too. He delights in making 'vroom vroom' noises when pushing her around town in the wheelchair. Recently he enjoyed weaving in and out of scaffolding poles erected all along one pavement making his favourite noise! And, in case anyone thinks that's all very well for someone who's young, the gentleman in question is 70 years old!

But what of those who can't share their laughter with their dependant? Is it impossible to keep one's humour then? Ruth didn't find it so although she does wish she had been able to share one particular incident with her dying father. She and her husband ran a busy pub and in order to be able to hear her father when he wanted help, they rigged up a bell. Late one night, as they were closing and people were leaving, two very drunk men came in demanding a drink. The situation looked like turning nasty when all of a sudden her father's bell rang out loud and long. One man jumped sky high, pushed his mate and said 'That's a ... fire bell!' With that they stumbled into the night. There were probably many times when that bell was a nuisance to Ruth when she was busy but the result of the bell, on that particular occasion, was the cause of great amusement long afterwards.

When the going gets even tougher one can still see the funny side of things. Joan had to do everything for her husband even when she had broken her ankle, although the nurses came frequently to care for him until she was more mobile. But on the first morning of their independence a problem arose as to how to give him his breakfast as she was still on crutches. She solved it by pouring his tea into a medicine bottle, wrapping a sandwich in a serviette and tucking both into her bra, thus allowing both hands free for the crutches. He enjoyed that meal and often referred to it laughingly as his 'bra breakfast'.

All the above are wonderful ways to overcome grief and loss. They can and do sustain but on their own they will always fall short of God's best for us. The third point is that, as we leave our period of mourning behind, we will not just be restored to cope and get by but that we can also receive God's joy. Perhaps this is one occasion where the Christian has that little more to offer the hurting carer.

The Psalmist David went through much despair and when we are feeling really low, his Psalms are a real comfort because he has put into words our deepest feelings and longings. But he moved on from these moments of despair, to moments of great joy and praise to God. In Psalm 30:5 he states: 'Weeping may tarry for the night, but joy comes with the morning.' The prophet Jeremiah also speaks of the fact that God will restore His people. 'I will turn their mourning into joy, I will comfort them, and give them gladness for sorrow.'

Wonderful assurances and promises but how do we accept and apply them to us when our circumstances remain the same and are not transformed in any dramatic way? The answer perhaps lies in the fact that true joy does not depend on circumstance. Yes, God does restore us but not necessarily by removing difficulties. Joy is not the same as happiness.

However good the above remedies are one cannot be sustained permanently by such things. 'The kingdom of heaven does not mean food and drink but righteousness and peace and joy in the Holy Spirit' (Romans 14:17). Such things are material and transient and bring happiness, which is good, but they will not yield the deep satisfying joy which the Holy Spirit gives. We can experience this only as we allow Him access to our lives so that our deepest sighs and longings can be dealt with.

Joy is something else and stands quite apart from happiness. It is knowing the Lord Jesus Christ and abiding in His love. It will involve giving ourselves to Him whatever may befall and whatever we may feel like. The gospel of John (chapter 15) explains how we can abide in Christ and His love and we have already spoken about this in the previous chapter.

But the good news is that He even offers us something extra to His love: 'These things have I spoken to you, that My joy may be in you, and that your joy may be full' (John 15:11). It is this deep joy which we can receive if we allow Him to come and abide. It is His joy, free for the taking, but we have to turn from our sorrow.

'My times are in Your hands' says the Psalmist (Ps 31:16) and when the time comes to move on we have to take it. When the time of mourning is over we have to take the positive step of being willing to change. Grief is an attitude but so is joy. This does not mean we have to work it up within ourselves. Joy is another fruit (or evidence) of the Spirit just as love is. It is God-given. But We have to be willing to receive His gift!

It is no good wallowing in self pity, as this will only result in depression and bitterness. It is not even sufficient to rely on our own positive methods. To be truly healed from our grief we have to look up as the Psalmist did and fix our gaze on the Lord God. Then, and only then, can we receive this wonderful joy which far outshines ordinary happiness.

People often ask me how I can experience such joy when not only is life hard but I also have to bear continuous and severe pain every minute of the day and night. The answer is I couldn't begin to do so by my own strength alone. It would purely be living for the happy times and being stoical ... neither of which I would be able to sustain for long. But 'The joy of the Lord is your strength' (Nehemiah 8:10) and this is what I've found.

Of course I fail and fix eyes back on myself from time to time but mostly there is a wonderful spring of joy welling up within me. It is totally irrational and unexplainable but nevertheless very real. It is there in the bad times as well as the good and has been with me for several years. Indeed, as I get to know God more and spend more time just turning to Him and communing with Him, I am discovering that this joy increases and this despite the fact that our circumstances are steadily worsening.

So if life seems really cruel and hard and the losses far outweigh the gains, please don't despair. Just give it all over to God and in due time He will restore and bring joy. It won't happen overnight and it involves a daily surrender of oneself to God but you will begin to experience it, just as we have, and see that His mercies are indeed 'New every morning'.

Chapter 8
CALM AMIDST THE STORM

'What's God playing at?' 'Why has this to happened to me?' 'How will I cope?' 'Where will it all end?' 'Who can I turn to?' 'When is God going to step in and help me?' All these questions and many others flood our minds and disturb our peace when disaster strikes or life becomes difficult.

Helen worries about what will happen to her mentally handicapped daughter when she is no longer able to care for her. Those who are cared for, myself included, worry about what will happen to them if their carer becomes ill or dies. Claire speaks of the mental strain and anxiety of caring for her mother who doesn't live with her - always worrying if she is alright and wondering why she doesn't answer the phone. She also speaks of a personal anxiety as to what effect the constant lifting will have on her, physically, in the long term. And so it can continue. Life can be so difficult and such a struggle that our minds are filled with anxiety. When one's emotions are also in a turmoil these worries become magnified and our peace is lost.

As a situation continues and worsens it is so easy to become bitter and resentful. Eileen has a very difficult time coping with a husband suffering from senile dementia. One can detect the underlying bitterness and resentment when she says, 'It's a cruel ending to a clean living and considerate gentleman.'

Envy of others creeps in too as does anger and frustration.

All this has happened to us - even as Christians. Whenever we took our eyes off God and focused on the circumstances we lost the peace which once was ours.

Those who don't really have a personal faith, as we had, often lose a kind of superficial peace. This is the peace which we all experience through absence of stress and a life of ease.

But, whatever kind of peace is lost, through whatever kind of circumstances that have befallen, the main question to ask and try to answer is;:'Can such peace be restored or even discovered for the first time even if the situation remains the same?'

God can give us an unexplainable peace ...
often without our asking

God is so good and loving to all His creation regardless of whether they acknowledge Him or not. When we are suddenly hit by a catastrophe, we are so often aware of an unexplainable sense of peace. This peace sustains us over the initial shock. At such a time we may not be able to think straight, let alone pray and yet this peaceful Presence surrounds and cushions us, we feel enveloped in warmth and protection and all the normal fears and anxieties cannot touch us. So many people have testified to this. Joan was aware of many people praying for her and puts it thus: 'It was like a blanket wrapped around me, sustaining me at all times.'

Some may not acknowledge a loving God behind such peace. Some may realize that, although they have no faith themselves, someone else's prayers have been upholding them and that God is hearing and answering.

This wonderful peace perhaps comes as no surprise to those of us with a personal faith and yet it is no less remarkable for that.

I can remember one such experience. It was almost nine years ago and yet it still remains vividly in my mind. After being extremely ill for about six weeks at home, I was finally admitted to a hospital in Manchester. We are not really Northerners and as Manchester is about a hundred miles south of us, I had never even been there. I arrived exhausted in an ambulance, frightened, alone and feeling very ill. I gradually settled in. My husband was able to visit me for a couple of hours or so on the weekend and this was the highlight of the week.

I can remember feeling so helpless and alone when everyone else had crowds of visitors each day. I didn't mind the lack of visitors as I felt too ill to bother anyway, but the worst thing was that I was so helpless. The nurses were so busy and one couldn't keep bothering them for all the little things, like straightening the bed or getting something out of reach. It was hard enough making sure I had a decent wash, my teeth cleaned and my hair combed! At the end of the week my allotted space would look as if a bomb had hit it and my husband spent a busy half hour sorting me out again.

The experience was enough to shatter and upset anyone, and yet at the end of three weeks another bombshell was dropped and again I felt so isolated. Although I was feeling much better, there was a limit to what could be done for me without surgery. Normally this would require a very long waiting period as it was not a question of life and death for me. However, one morning a surgeon appeared and said they had had a cancellation and could operate within a few days but they would need my answer very soon. I had never had major surgery before and although the success rate was good and the operation would be done by a top surgeon, there were risks and I was so far away from home. My husband would not be able to visit before the operation and so, apart from one or two calls (have you ever tried to discuss anything long distance on a pay phone?) the decision had to be mine.

I made my decision and agreed to have the surgery done. It was then I experienced the most incredible peace. The day before the operation I would have normally been terrified and yet I wasn't. I certainly would have wanted my husband around to visit (or even anyone) but this was not possible. Yet I can remember chatting and laughing all day. This was not put on as I also ate well. I remember munching a bag of crisps with my last drink. That night I had a lovely peaceful sleep without any medication. One might be able to manufacture false calm and unconcern by one's attitude and mask one's deepest fears but one is not usually able to eat and sleep normally as well!

The day dawned and this incredible peace remained all through the preparations. I don't think I really needed the pre-operation sedative. I remained very alert and very calm right until the final knockout jab and countdown. Even afterwards, I was so alert and calm. I recall coming round in a recovery room and being one of a row of patients on stretchers. The nurse looked at me and said 'This one can go back now. She's on Ward H1.' And I calmly replied 'No, I'm on Ward H2.'

For the next few days this unbelievable peace enveloped me. I was not in a tired stupor but very alert and indeed was soon put to work with physiotherapists etc. I also know it wasn't an imagined peace because some two or three weeks later one of the nurses confided, 'We couldn't understand how calm you could be, especially just before the operation. Most people are really scared.'

Such experiences are really very hard to describe and very hard to imagine if you have not had them yourself. It has happened to me on several occasions since and is certainly not diminished by being repeated. However, such things seem to be a special endowment of God's grace when we are in particular need and cannot be conjured up to order, even by prayer. Indeed sometimes they occur without prayer or faith. He knows our need and when we are totally helpless and dependent He supplies it.

This peace is also ours to receive for the asking

About six months later, the whole operation needed to be repeated on another part of my anatomy. This time it was planned and we were able to make suitable arrangements concerning the children, thus enabling my husband to drive me to hospital and stay until the evening which meant I was only alone for the day before my operation and this was a very busy day of preparation anyway. I expected the same peace. I knew lots of people were praying for me. The doctors and nurses were no longer strangers. I had made arrangements for people living in the Manchester area to visit me after the operation. This time I knew exactly what the stay in hospital entailed and, after all, it is often fear of the unknown which unsettles our well-being. Yet the peace alluded me.

I panicked and cried my eyes out when my husband left. I felt fearful as I was prepared for surgery the next morning and was glad to get my pre-med. I did not experience the same alertness this time (perhaps the anaesthetic was different) and felt quite off for a day or so afterwards.

So what does this mean? Can we not expect God's peace when we ask for it? Is it some arbitrary thing which we have no control over? If so, we might as well not bother to pray for it. Well, yes, I feel this special kind of peace is often bestowed in an almost arbitrary manner. It is certainly nothing we have done to deserve and God seems to bestow it on who He will, as a measure of His grace and mercy, in much the same way as He bestows many of His other blessings.

I didn't feel this very special peace the second time round, but I'm sure the fault lay with me, and that God allowed it in order to show me the difference between being totally helpless and dependent on Him and being rather organised and self sufficient, and feeling we had got the whole situation under our control and that the bestowal of His peace was just all a part of my organised plans and something to be expected almost without consulting Him.

The circumstances were almost identical and it should have been easier the second time. But that did not mean He had withdrawn from me. I'm sure God's peace was there, readily available, had I not panicked and taken my eyes from Him. Yes, He can step in in a special way without us doing anything but generally speaking He does not force Himself on us and we usually have to respond by receiving whatever it is He offers; in this case, His peace.

So how can we receive this peace?

God is peace

Jesus is the Prince of Peace (Isaiah 9:6) and promises us His peace. He said to His disciples that He would leave His peace with them. It would not be

a natural peace brought about through absence of difficulties and a life of ease but rather a supernatural one, not dependent on circumstances. 'Peace I will leave with you; my peace I give to you; not as the world gives do I give to you. Let not your hearts be troubled, neither let them be afraid' (John 14:27).

Because of our right relationship with God through the sacrifice of Jesus we have his peace. His love 'has been poured into our hearts' enabling us to rejoice and have hope even in the midst of our sufferings (Romans 5:1-5). We have access to God and His peace. It is freely available to us. It is another fruit (or evidence) of the Spirit and similar to joy and love which are very much dependent on our attitude and willingness to receive them.

Look to God
We first have to fix our eyes on God and away from ourselves and our circumstances. Then He is able to bring us His peace. 'Thou dost keep Him in perfect peace, whose mind is stayed on thee, because he trusts in thee' (Isaiah 26:3).

Allow God to give us His peace
We then have to allow Him to meet our need in whatever way He chooses. Again this is an act of will. The verse from John's gospel, which has already been quoted, says don't *let* your hearts be troubled or afraid. Another verse taken from the letter the apostle Paul wrote to the church at Colossae says: '*Let* the peace of Christ rule in your hearts' (Colossians 3:15).

When we do this and are no longer anxious but instead we will find that His peace floods in. 'Rejoice.... The Lord is at hand. Have no anxiety about anything, but in everything by prayer and supplication with thanksgiving let your requests be made known to God. And the peace of God which passes all understanding, will keep your hearts and minds in Christ Jesus,' says Paul again, but this time to the Philippian church (Phil 4:7).

Apart from the very special occasions, this type of peace has been our experience over the past fourteen years. It has sustained us and always been there in the most dark and bleak times. I know it is the experience of others too. Mary confided that they live one day at a time 'trusting it all to God for tomorrow - even if it all went wrong today.'

In case some people think this is all very glib and easy for me to say and that they don't have our sort of faith or their circumstances are far worse than ours, I would like to share that such peace has not always been easy to find. Our own doubts and fears have crept in and threatened to consume. These have been the depressing times when God has seemed a million miles away and our circumstances have taken over. They have been the times of tears and worry, bitterness and resentment, anger and frustration. They have been the times when our grief and loss have filled our minds and we have been able to see little good in anything. They have always been the times when we have taken our eyes off God and started looking inward.

I believe such times were more prevalent in the early years of my illness when we had not had time to grieve or come to terms with things and when we had not had all the experience we have now of knowing God's love and peace right in the middle of it all.

We had not had the chance to trust Him in the way we have to do all the time now nor the wealth of evidence to show us how He has always been there and never failed us. We have learned to trust and depend on Him because there is really nothing else to put our trust in. When you come to the end of yourself then you can discover that He was there all the time and that He has your best interests at heart and when you entrust yourself to Him, His contentment and peace are just always available. Very little flusters and disturbs us now. Indeed, it is usually the silly little things which we are not prepared for.

But that is the present and there are many lessons to be learned from the past. When one's peace is shattered it is so easy for resentment and bitterness to build up and take root and if this has happened it needs dealing with if one's peace and right relationship with God is to be restored. This was my experience.

We had been married two years, both had good jobs and had been able to furnish and start buying our own house. We were both keen Christians and now to crown our happiness I had just become pregnant. God was really good and everything was going according to plan (our plan that is).

We didn't realise the self centred lives we were leading at the time because we always prayed and committed everything to God and truly believed we were in His will. Perhaps we were. I can't honestly say because I don't think we allowed any listening space to find out. It is easy to assume that we are in His will because everything is going smoothly. We pray and expect God to bless our schemes and plans and be manipulated and manoeuvred into allowing us to plan the direction of our lives and yet put a God-label on them because, after all, we have consulted Him! Many Christians spend their lives in this way and it is not wrong. We were not being deliberately disobedient and we were giving our time and energies to Him. However, I believe He had something more in store for us which we could never have experienced in this life of ease.

I didn't know this at the time and some three months later our world was shattered never to be the same again. I lost the baby and whilst still in hospital I noticed my thumbs felt a bit stiff and painful. I took the loss of the baby very hard but I didn't allow myself time to grieve openly. I thought it peculiar to feel such grief for a child which had never actually lived and so I stifled it. I now think quite differently about the unborn child and see such grief as normal and natural. But I was young and there was no one to share it with, or so I felt.

I went back to work but the rest of my body began to be affected in the same way as my thumbs until there was scarcely anywhere unaffected and free from pain. At the same time I could not go near women with babies.

I remember a holiday that summer in Bournemouth when I couldn't bear to go on the beach because there I would be surrounded by children. My husband must have had quite a puzzling holiday being directed to the garden or peace and quiet of the New Forest. It was whilst on this holiday that we bought a dinghy, with the view of taking my mind off things.

The doctors could find nothing wrong with me at this stage and believing it all to be psychological advised me to have another baby as soon as possible. But one cannot escape with a dinghy or another baby and I was building up resentments.

They were resentments against the doctor for allowing the miscarriage to occur and resentments against anyone with a baby or toddler. This was resentment touched with real anger against God. Neither Chris nor I are angry people. Indeed, we are extremely placid but the question of 'Why, why, why have you let all this happen to us' was never far away.

I remember one woman in particular who went to the same home Bible-study group. She had three children and for some reason I singled her out and deep within always felt 'it's alright for you, you've got everything.'

Actually, God taught me a valuable lesson through that too because a little while later she contracted cancer and died, leaving a husband and three young children. I felt awful but it taught me never to envy again and never to look at others and say 'it's not fair'. Only God can see the end from the beginning and it's not our role.

It is our role to accept ourselves and the place where God has placed us. We are unique and only entrusted with what is best for us. To be in that place and accept it is true peace, but again it took years to appreciate fully.

Unbeknown to me, Chris was undergoing similar sorts of battles. He admits to having an 'it's not fair' attitude for years. He recalls one occasion in particular when he returned home from a school fete, feeling sick to the stomach, having spent the entire time observing normal family groups and couples strolling happily about.

In both our cases we needed to recognise these areas of resentment, bitterness and anger and to repent of (or turn away from) them. As we experienced God's forgiveness His peace was able to flow once more.

But it didn't happen overnight. We received it gradually over a period of years. Having dealt with the bitterness and resentment and made sure that there were no other areas in our lives, revealed to us by the Holy Spirit, which also needed putting right, we now needed to accept the situation.

It is so easy to fret and struggle and not give everything over to God, because we are not willing to trust that He is in control of the situation and has our best interests at heart. It is so much more comfortable to feel we have an element of control over our lives and it is sad that it is often only in moments of utter desperation, when we admit we can do nothing, that we are willing to give up. What a lot of pain we would save ourselves if this was our first resort instead of our last!

However, it was as we let go and looked up that we began to see things from a different perspective. God began to show us what His heart and mind were in the matter. It was painful. We didn't always like what we heard. But gradually, as we have started to see things from His angle (which, after all, is an eternal perspective, not a temporal one) we were able to look up and beyond and His peace flooded in.

Philippians 4:11 has been a very meaningful verse to me ever since I began my quest for peace and sought His forgiveness all those years ago. But I am still learning the meaning of ' being content in whatever state I am' and that 'knowing Christ' surpasses everything else (Philippians 3:8).

I am aware that what I say may not be acceptable in some circles. To some it would be seen as an extreme form of escapism in order to be able to cope and have peace of mind. All I can say is that it is not. It is far harder to face up to things and accept them than it is to try and escape in other ways. I have tried. I know what it was like being hooked on painkillers and craving the feeling of wooziness they brought rather than face the pain (which, incidentally, they could not quench). Whenever I have striven and struggled and fought I have known torment in body and spirit. But the glorious alternative has been wonderful peace even in the midst of intense suffering.

I am also aware that others would say that it is not God's will for us to be in the situation we are and that to accept it is wrong. But there is a difference in accepting a situation when we have not sought God over it, to doing so, when we have. We don't pretend to understand it all or have all the answers. Neither do we feel life is always fair. God is not fair. He treats us all differently and has different plans for each one of us but it is enough to know that He is always just.

When we give our lives to God we have to be prepared for the cost. There will always be one and the more we want to move on with Him, the higher it will be, in order for His work to be fully accomplished in us. The cosy message preached by some about 'coming to Christ and He will solve all your problems' is just not true and does so much more harm than good. Instead, I feel it should be 'Come to Christ. He may not remove all your problems. He doesn't send them but He may allow them in order to make you into the person He wants you to be. Rest assured that this way may not be easy but it puts you back into a wonderful relationship with Him which far surpasses any peace, joy or contentment you'll find anywhere else! The joy of knowing God will far transcend the difficulties and the rest for the soul, which one finds, is peace indeed.'

We have always wanted to know God in a very deep way and to give ourselves completely to Him. For us, at this time, the cost is the privilege of being allowed to suffer for Him. For others it will be something quite different and may well be far less severe and long-lasting. It isn't that He sends bad things along in order to whip us into shape. It is rather that sometimes He permits them to continue for in so doing He can bring such good from them if only we let Him.

Having spent many years in asking God to remove our problems and ease our burdens, it is only now that we are beginning to receive and accept His purpose for our lives and to know that we are right where He wants us for the time being. Such knowledge brings real peace, and we are beginning to understand Paul (who had suffered much) when he declared that he counted everything else loss compared with gaining Christ. It may sound like 'pie in the sky' and it is impossible to explain, but it works. However hard your life may be as a carer, if that is truly what God has called you to be, then accept it and wait for His peace to flood your being!

Chapter 9
WITH STRENGTH RENEWED

"Daaaddyyy!" "Chriiss!" seem to be the frequent cries in our household and isn't it strange that they almost always occur just as my husband eases himself into an armchair for a five minute break! Back to work and just in the middle of it all the telephone or doorbell rings!

Being a carer can be very tiring. My husband's day usually begins at 6.50 am when the alarm goes off. At 9.15 am there is a momentary breather before he begins the day's work proper. All that happens in the previous two hours or so is mere routine; the daily round of getting himself up, making breakfast, seeing two children off to school, clearing the breakfast things, doing the beds and finally getting me up. He's lucky! The boys do help with the chores and I am able to supervise from my bed ... chivvying the boys along, listening to spellings or French vocabulary, having a cuddle and 'quiet time' with both of them. At 9.15 am (or 9.00 am if we really put our skates on and perhaps do some overnight preparation) we are ready to face the world should someone call or we have to attend an early appointment.

The same thing happens all day long. Even with the boys at school there are still two lots of everything to do. There are two coats to put on if we go out, two people's personal hygiene to see to and so on. As well as this he has to do all the jobs normally shared by two.

Of course, there are spare moments in the day before the boys return but these are usually filled by catching up on extra jobs. It may be DIY, gardening or shopping. Sometimes it involves doing something for someone else or church.

When the boys arrive home it's all systems go again until at least 9.00 pm when we're all in bed. But as the children get older even this alters and often Chris has scarcely sat down before his own bedtime.

We are not grumbling, nor do we see our situation as unique. There must be many others for whom this sort of day is fairly typical and probably far worse. At least not all my husband's tasks are thankless and joyless by any means and much of it is the result of the responsibilities and ties that marriage and rearing a family bring. There are bonuses too. On a fine day we can sometimes just drop everything and take a morning or afternoon off.

Many other people also lead very busy lives and get very tired. Perhaps one subtle difference, though, is that much of this is a result of their own choosing. We can choose to be ambitious and lead demanding work lives, putting in long and exhausting hours. Whether the choice comes from dedication to a calling like a doctor, nurse or pastor or perhaps from more selfish reasons is immaterial. The important point is that there is an element of choice in most life-styles.

We can also choose to take on busy social lives. We can even choose to fill our time being busy for God. We can often choose to be working Mums. Some people can never just 'be' and always have to fill each moment of the day with something. It can be a calling or just plain escapism. If such people are exhausted perhaps it is time for them to examine their priorities and see what they can let go of and indeed what would be best for them to release.

However, some people - carers, single parents or Mums with large families - do not have such a choice to make unless they choose to opt out and run away. They have to keep going whatever and cannot afford the time to be ill, even if only for a few days! Is it possible to avoid the exhaustion and stress such a way of life may unavoidably bring?

We have discovered two solutions. The first is spiritual and needs to be put first:

1. We need to receive the strength which is available from God

Some people do seem to have a lot to bear and do spend most of their lives in sacrificial giving to others. They are often in danger of wearing themselves out in the process if they are not able or willing to fix their gaze higher than themselves and draw on the strength so freely offered by God. But how can we be sure He can supply our need and help us?

Recognise that God understands
God always points us to His Son. Jesus has been there before us and doesn't ask more from us than we can do. He doesn't give us anything that He himself has not experienced either. He was often weary. He travelled on

long, hot and dusty journeys. After one such journey, He sat down wearily by a well and asked a woman for water and then proceeded to minister to her, tired though He must have been.

Everywhere Jesus went the crowds flocked to Him demanding His attention and that their needs be met. He crossed Lake Galilee and the crowds followed. Later He went up into the hills with His disciples to sit down and rest. Still the multitude pursued Him. In the same chapter we read that on another occasion the crowds went searching for Him and eventually went after Him in boats. This sort of thing was happening all the time. So who better to understand our weariness.

Recognise that God is never too weary to answer a cry for help and strength
Jesus never turned anyone away and because He has experienced such weariness Himself, He is able to offer us His strength to cope. If we come to Him He can give us His rest and our burdens will be lightened (Matthew 11:28,29). The almighty God never tires or grows weary and if we wait on Him our strength will be renewed. We will 'Mount up with wings like eagles'. We will 'Run and not be weary, walk and not be faint' (Isaiah 40:28-31). What beautiful, encouraging words. If we really take them to heart and respond to them, we can have victory over the most stressful and exhausting situations.

We have seen how we can receive God's love, joy and peace. Once again, we need to respond and deliberately and consciously be willing to receive from Him. But this time to receive His strength.

2. We can also help ourselves
If we are making our lives more stressful by our life-style or by our own stubbornness in not seeking help and try and modify the situation, it is hardly surprising if we do not experience the strength God can give us. He cannot work in us if we are not willing to change our attitudes which could so easily be the underlying cause of our weariness.

Whenever we have insisted on carrying on, reliant on our own strength, pressure and stress have naturally built up and we have become even more tired than we would have been.

The first priority has always been to let go and allow God to control the situation, but the next step has been to look at our life-style and see how it can be adapted to be the least tiring possible.

Ideally, both carer and dependant need to do this together, wherever possible, as there needs to be give and take on both sides. Nobody should be expected to carry the burden of continual care unaided. Everyone needs a break. For a full-time carer who looks after someone needing constant supervision this is obviously a real problem. What practical ways can this be achieved?

Take a break for a few days
It may never be possible to take a break for as much as a day or so without careful planning. Naturally, in an emergency the person cared for will have to be taken into care and this will probably mean hospital or a nursing home which provides nursing care. However, planned breaks can be arranged. (The chapter on help from the State will give more details of what respite care is available).

This seems such an obvious solution and those who take advantage of it speak of the benefits. Eileen says 'There is no way one can entertain company or be sure of keeping an appointment. I am truly thankful that the hospital have now arranged a fortnight's respite in every ten weeks so that I can get a thorough sleep, can visit my son and give our flat a good clean because the one gift my husband still has is acute hearing. He can hear me turning over pages in the next room and shouts in protest at the noise of a vacuum cleaner, the typewriter in the flat above, or me washing the dishes.'

* Take a break - even if you feel guilty at doing so. Many carers feel guilty at taking such a break. Helen feels guilty at leaving her mentally handicapped daughter in a home for the occasional weekend or week but she does it. This means a break not only for her but the rest of the family too. They can do things together as a 'normal' family. Her eight year-old daughter is able have her parents to herself and some of her needs are met for a change.

* Take a break - even if your dependant is awkward and difficult about it. Some dependants can make the situation even worse by being difficult. For several years Jackie's grandmother lived with her and her husband. She had to do everything for her and with two small children as well they obviously needed breaks. The social worker arranged for Gran to go into a home for two weeks every summer so that they could have a family holiday. This was lovely but was always tinged with a feeling of guilt because Gran did not like them to leave her. She would start to cry and wish she were dead so that she wouldn't be such a burden. But, however hard it was to do, they had their holiday and benefited.

* Take a break - do not be tempted to keep going. Some carers are not so sensible and just carry on. Kathleen tells of her sister who took over her job of caring for her mother when she herself became disabled. Friends offered to stay with her mother while her sister took a break. But her mother wouldn't have it. Instead of insisting, her sister kept going until she eventually suffered a nervous breakdown. The mother was then taken into permanent care. Perhaps if they had both been more sensible such a situation would never have arisen.

I can sympathise with the dependants. The thought of respite care does not appeal to me. There is no place like home when one is unwell and, unfortunately, I'm not just disabled but also unwell. But recently I sampled it for myself for a few weeks. My husband had a hernia. He needed it seeing to and was not able to lift me properly for three months afterwards. Once he had recovered from the operation we were able to rely on friends and district nurses to help with the lifting and he coped in all the other ways as usual. But it still meant I needed to go into respite care for three weeks. It was very tempting to be 'difficult' and wallow in self pity. Perhaps I could have been excused for doing so a little because I knew that the change in routines would affect me adversely and that I wasn't just being selfish. Indeed, I admit to succumbing to a few miserable hours. But I had to put him first. He does so much for me. It was not exactly a pleasant prospect for him and I could have made it ten times worse. The poor dear is not even able to be unwell in peace. With God's help I was able to commit the whole situation to Him and know that even if I couldn't look forward to it, He would be with us both through it and would even bring good out of it and, of course, this was the case.

Take a short, regular break

Most people could manage a break for an hour or two a week and there are many schemes, both voluntary and also those run by the state which can come to our aid. Perhaps there is a friend or member of one's family who can help out in order to make this possible.

* Co-operation - makes it possible. That Chris needs breaks is obvious to me but I still need to be open in making it work. This is another area where I could become difficult. It is so easy to become very demanding and introverted but I have to make a conscious effort to put him first just as he does for me nearly every moment of the day. It requires sacrifice and it may not be a pleasant proposition but I must be willing to make it happen. We have tried to discuss and pray together about what kind of break would be most edifying and also what would be possible to maintain on a regular basis.

Chris likes to get away from it all one morning a week. He feels the need to be alone and also to get some exercise as we of necessity usually travel everywhere by car. Living on the edge of the Lake District and having so much beauty right on our doorstep, the obvious solution for him is to go walking. Buying a pair of boots and fixing a time was the easy part! We then had to look at all the ways to make it happen.

* Practical planning - makes it possible. On a purely practical level we needed to make me as independent as possible so that Chris was able to be released. We will be discussing all the advice and practical help that is available in a later chapter but as far as we were concerned we needed to provide me with some mobility and also some means of contacting the outside world in an emergency. This has meant an electric wheelchair and a portable phone and with these I am able to be left for a couple of hours. I can't pretend I enjoy the thought of having to sit in the same chair for two or three hours and I feel a bit insecure on my own but it is possible and I can see how very important it is to give Chris a regular break. I have a word processor and prepare our weekly church newsletter so I take the opportunity of doing it then and the time flies by.

We have just had our house adapted and now I am even more independent with a ramp giving access to the outside of the house and also a remote controlled back door with which I can not only to let myself in and out but also open the door to visitors.

The most difficult problem to overcome has been that of going to the toilet. Our solution is not ideal and I can't say it appeals to me but I have had to be willing to be treated as incontinent when he is out. If the time came, I suppose we would have to have a nurse to come and be with me. Friends and family, however willing, are not really able to deal with this. I cannot just be treated as a 'sack of coal' and humped about; I am in too much pain for that and, if I am honest, I would prefer a professional person to deal with such intimate things anyway.

However, we make use of help in other ways. I could be left for three hours I suppose but we have a better arrangement. Once a week we go to my mother-in-law for lunch and on another day she comes to us. It has been an arrangement of some longstanding and suits us all. The day we go to Mum's, my husband does the cleaning and is grateful not to have to get dinner as well. The day she comes to us is her shopping day and the same applies. With a little thought we have adapted this arrangement and she comes an hour earlier than necessary in order to see that I am OK., make us both a cuppa and put the already-prepared dinner on. The arrangement suits us all admirably and a way has been found round a potentially impossible situation.

On advice from the doctor, during a particularly traumatic time, Joan used her 'break period' to take up a new hobby. She enrolled in a class at the local college and took up drawing and painting. She found a love and aptitude for it and was delighted by the encouragement of her friends who were kind and considerate and made house room for her pictures.

* Well worth it. Having been prepared to 'give a bit', I have discovered (as I always do) that the sacrifice is more than made up for. Chris returns home fresh and ready to carry on for another week and I have accomplished something too. The break from each other is equally beneficial and helps us to maintain a degree of independence, however brief, in lives which are far more intricately bound together than is usual.

Special treats

* Co-operation once again! Carers need special treats and dependants need to be willing to allow them to happen. I try to allow Chris special treats from time to time. These would probably not be considered as 'treats' by most people as they are just a normal, fairly frequent happening but, for him, they can usually only take place once a year or even once every two years and so they are treats indeed! His favourite treat is to attend a country and western concert every December.

Kathleen's experience was not so happy. Before her sister took over the care of her mother, Kathleen took her mother with them on a family holiday. Just for once she and her husband wanted an evening to themselves so they asked her mother if she would be willing to stay in with their daughter (then about 14 years old). But her mother didn't want to be left. They explained they weren't taking the car but going for a walk. Normally her mother wouldn't walk far and this was a long walk they had planned. But not only did her mother manage it she was in front all the way! She could not even allow them an occasional treat. No wonder her poor sister had a breakdown a few years later when her mother needed more care!

* Careful planning once again. First and foremost for us is my willingness to be treated as incontinent. We then have to find a suitable sitter for myself and the children. We have one or two past helpers who more than fit the bill as they not only know the children well, but also me, and are able to take over and be in charge whilst I am in bed and at the same time do not wear me out! They lead very busy lives themselves and we do not like to put upon them too often, so sometimes a shorter outing means being willing to just have someone 'on call'. Knowing they are only a phone call away and having my cordless phone within reach and also a smoke detector installed makes this possible. It is not very pleasant to feel trapped in bed knowing Chris is not on hand to lift me out in an emergency, but it is more than worth it to see the pleasure and almost childish joy such a treat affords.

* Well worth it once again! Chris returns from his treat refreshed and I have benefited too. I have had the treat of having a very dear friend to myself all evening. It has been a time of joy in just chatting and sharing together. It may have taken quite a lot out of me and mean I need to rest up for a few days afterwards but when one has seldom had any evening activity for several years it is quite stimulating.

Even the most careful planning is brought to nought sometimes. There are times when I am just too ill to release Chris. Sometimes it coincides with his morning walk ... it may be just an off day and I'm usually better the next but his walk has to be cancelled. At other times there has been a really dark patch and we have both been pretty housebound for several months. Occasionally I have an unavoidable appointment which comes on the wrong day. Add to this the days when he has had to cancel through the normal course of events: the boys are off school, the weather is awful, he doesn't feel well, he is busy with something else etc. and you can see that it can be frustrating. However, Chris just seems to be able to put it behind him and carry on as before. This is essential however disappointed and annoyed he must feel. I think having a good relationship and a lot of give and take on both sides makes it easier to bear. I'm sure he prays about it too and is learning to take his disappointments to God.

Have time alone

Outings on his own are few and precious but it is also important for Chris to have time on his own at home. Once again this is where I can play my part. It's so easy to keep discovering more jobs needing to be done. When the house is quiet and Chris is alone doing something how often have I called him away to see to me. Sometimes it is inevitable of course but there must have been many times when it wasn't really necessary. Perhaps I dropped something and wanted it retrieved or perhaps I wanted the television on and so I would call out and interrupt. I am learning to see how necessary my demands are before I trouble him and even if I have to be patient and frustrated while I wait, I think it's important sometimes to do just that and put him first.

It can have it's funny side too. I have two wheelchairs; one is electric, the other pushed by someone else. Chris gets confused sometimes and will leave me staring at a wall for a while, go off into the garden to do a job and quite forget that I'm immobile in the push-only chair. Even I get confused and remain motionless when in the electric one! It is good to have a sense of humour and be able to see the funny side instead of getting annoyed and impatient with each other.

It would be so easy to be on top of each other and this is wrong too. During the day I no longer follow Chris round as I once did. He needs to be able to get on in his own way. I have needed other activities and God has very graciously provided me with some and shown me areas where He wants to use me. Okay, I'll always be a Mum and housewife in my mind but for now these roles have been relinquished in any active and practical sense and I'm finding that other outlets, although perhaps not of my own choosing, have been chosen by a loving God and are absolutely right. As well as allowing me to do something in my Christian service, they also keep me occupied and give us a break from each other. Organising and writing are the two main ways I keep busy and out of Chris's way when he is doing the chores. Then we are ready to spend time together at home or go out, with friends or to meetings.

Keep your own friends
We need our own friends too and try not to always stay in the same room when someone has called to see only one of us. Actually, if someone calls for me, it is a good opportunity for Chris to be released to go and do something else, knowing someone is around to keep an eye on me. People have a habit of turning up at appropriate moments! Is it just coincidence I wonder or does it have something to do with giving the day over to God?

Maintain hobbies and interests at home
I must let Chris have his hobbies and interests too. For his part, he has been wonderful in adapting them to our situation and finds plenty to do when he gets time but I must let him. I have to go to bed early. When I am in bed it would be wrong to expect him to give up the rest of his evening entertaining me. There are times when we spend our evenings together of course. Perhaps he will come to bed early too and we will listen to the radio or a cassette. But he also needs his snatched half hours to himself sometimes to work at his hobbies or have a time alone with God or just sit in a chair and do nothing! He may not be able to go out much but from time to time he has a friend round to play trains or even just for coffee.

Bring people to the home
We are not able to go out together in the evening. As we can't get to evening meetings, where possible, we try to arrange to have them come to us. People are now well used to arriving for a meeting at eight o' clock and seeing no sign of me but are happy that at least Chris can join in.

Get enough rest

All these practical solutions are ways of ensuring one doesn't get too tired and weary. It helps keep a freshness and vitality in the relationship too. But if a carer is still getting very tired it is good to look at just how much rest one is getting.

* Sleep when the dependant sleeps. If you're worn out it may be necessary to sleep when the dependant sleeps. What is the point of staying up late and then having disturbed and difficult nights? It's good to take breaks from time to time but instead of using them for outings or indulging in hobbies, sometimes it would make more sense to go and have a sleep. If a dependant takes a rest in the daytime it can be a jolly good chance to catch up on jobs or have a bit of time to oneself, but a rest once in a while may be far more important. A lot of people would feel guilty about doing this but there is not reason why not if it's going to enable you to feel refreshed and ready to carry on again.

Chris, more or less, keeps to my hours as there are often disturbed nights as well as the busy days. I may go to bed anytime between five and eight o' clock but I'm usually ready for sleep by ten. Partly because of disturbing me, Chris obliged and started coming to bed by this time but now we find it quite sensible anyway. There are later nights, of course, but generally speaking, keeping such hours means he is ready to start the day early, and there is no chance of a lie-in with me or the boys!

* Ask for outside help. Another alternative is to consider asking for help either with the housework or perhaps to mind your dependant just so that you can have a sleep. There are other ways of relaxing too, perhaps a nice hot bath and time to pamper oneself would do much to restore ones aching, tired limbs or over-active mind. However you choose to spend your 'time off' it is wise to remember that these areas are vital too. It does seem to be that mutual co-operation and respect go a long way to solving all these problems more easily. I know from talking to others in similar situations that these are real problem areas and I feel so sad for people who are not able to be open and honest with each other. So often the desire not to hurt the other person and the feeling that they won't understand or be able to adapt, prevents this from happening. But one doesn't have to make radical changes. Just a little give and take can work wonders as we have discovered.

Even if this co-operation is not always possible there are other ways around the problem. The dependant may be unhelpful and the situation may seem impossible but the carer must make every effort to find solutions to give himself a break. At times it may mean insisting on it, however cruel and unkind it seems. It is for the good of both of you. Not so easy when one is already tired and overwrought and it just doesn't seem worth the hassle. But it is!

Even though help from other sources is not always ideal or easy to obtain it can usually be found and can relieve a little at the very least.

Ultimately one's own attitude with God can remove a lot of unnecessary stress and fatigue. He can change attitudes. Just as we can receive the love, joy and peace of God we can also receive his strength, even if the circumstances don't change. As Wendy says 'I did get physically tired (but I could cope with that) but not "fed up" tired!'

Chapter 10
LONELY YET NEVER ALONE

'We often try and masquerade as a "normal" family,' says Helen who finds ordinary things like shopping, taking a holiday and attending meetings a bit of an ordeal. 'We are entitled to have a disabled sticker on our car but so far we have managed to avoid advertising the fact that we have problems. I am a supply teacher and I often encounter rude children. It would give them even more ammunition to throw at me if I arrived in a car with a disabled badge!'

Life can be extremely lonely for a carer not just because it is difficult to get out and meet people but also because of feeling totally isolated even when amongst people. The actual situation cuts one off from normal, everyday life and it is not so easy to mix and join in with outside activities. This in turn makes one start to feel different and unable to communicate and relate to others. It can become a vicious circle. It is so easy to become introverted and withdrawn, feeling nothing can be done about the situation and getting so wrapped up in it that it is hard to shake off the lethargy it can bring. Sometimes of course people feel just too worn out and depressed to even try and mix with others and feel that all the effort involved is just not worth it.

Many carers, particularly those who have suddenly had illness, handicap, or disability inflicted on them and are struggling to come to terms with all the changes in their relationships and lifestyle, have discovered that friends and family, unable to cope, desert them completely. It seems a particular problem when the one being cared for suffers from a mental problem.

When Susan's husband returned from hospital, after six weeks, he was a completely different person. 'There he was swearing at whatever or whoever came his way and not recognising the fact either. From day one back home, friends and family disappeared overnight. And they have never returned.'

Gladys describes an experience which happened some time ago but one which obviously remains vivid in her memory: 'The worst part was the loneliness. People shun madness and my parents' friends (and mine) said it was too distressing to see them. Apart from going to work, I did not go out for six years except one evening when I bribed one of the helpers to stay on to enable me to go into London to buy underclothes as mine were in shreds.' Gladys took over from the paid helpers every day from 5 pm until 7.30 am the next morning. 'I had no one to talk to,' she says, 'I couldn't carry on a conversation with my parents. They talked 'scribble' night after night. It was hell.'

Sometimes the isolation is made harder to bear by well-meaning, insincere people. They promise much and deliver little. Some say how much they are thinking of you but never show it in any concrete or practical form.

Laura, who has a physically handicapped child, recounted to me how alone she felt during one period of her life. Her son had had an operation and was totally housebound for several weeks, and so she was as well. Many Christians told her how they were thinking of them and praying for them but only two people visited her during the entire time. One was obviously ill at ease and only stayed a few minutes making an excuse for a quick getaway. The other travelled from afar and spent a long time with them but never once asked how she was feeling.

At least the two who had visited had tried to show they cared, even if they had got it wrong. But if people do not really care or perhaps don't have the time to show it in practical ways then it would be better if they didn't make statements they don't really mean or promises they cannot fulfil. It can do more harm than good and increase the isolation rather than relieve it.

But it does no good to dwell on the failings of others. I only mentioned it to encourage would-be friends and helpers of carers to be honest and sincere with them. Ultimately they are answerable to God themselves for their behaviour and to dwell on such things only makes us bitter and resentful. Unfortunately, the isolation and loneliness makes one more prone to introversion and it is easy to let such things irritate and occupy our minds.

Perhaps it is better to turn to some solutions to the problem. We have discovered three main areas which can help.

1. God is always with us

Never really alone
However lonely, isolated, cut off and alone we feel it is good to remember we can never be really alone. Psalm 139 is a wonderful psalm which shows us that we can never be removed from the presence of God. He knows all about us from the time we were conceived in our mother's womb and is always with us and understands everything about us. 'If I ascend to heaven, Thou art there! If I make my bed in Sheol, Thou art there! If I take the wings of the morning and dwell in the uttermost parts of the sea, even there Thy hand shall lead me and Thy right hand shall hold me' (Psalm 139:8-10).

We can be God's friends
Because God is always with us and wants us to know and love His presence, He sent Jesus to make this possible and to restore the relationship broken through sin. 'Emmanuel', one of the names given to Jesus, means 'God with us' and so He is. 'At one time you were far away from God and were His enemies because of the evil things you did and thought. But now, by means of the physical death of His Son, God has made you His friends, in order to bring you, holy, pure and faultless into His presence' (Colossians 1:21,22).

When Jesus was living on the earth as man He knew God the Father had not left Him alone: John 8:29 says 'And He who has sent me is with me; He has not left me alone.' He also knew that, ultimately, He could not rely on His disciples to stand by Him, however close they had been to Him and said you 'will be scattered and ... leave Me alone; yet I am not alone, for the Father is with Me.' (John 16:32).

Jesus understands our aloneness
Although Jesus knew He was not alone, there must have been many times in His life when He felt so. He told a would-be disciple that: 'Foxes have holes, and birds of the air have nests; but the Son of man has nowhere to lay His head.' He spent forty days alone in the wilderness and was tempted by the devil and yet at the end of this time we read that 'Angels came and ministered to Him' (Matthew 3:11). God had not deserted Him.

Ultimately though, He had to take the way of the cross and it was here that for a brief period God the Father did leave Him. Jesus took our sins and the punishment for them upon Himself. But God is holy and righteous. He cannot look on sin, and so when Jesus was on the cross He cried out, 'My God, my God, why hast Thou forsaken me?'

But because Jesus took our sin on Himself, we need never be cut off from God again by sin. Indeed, we can now be called God's children (1 John 3:1,2). He delights in this relationship and longs that we may all experience it.

After His death, Jesus returned to His Father in heaven. He would resume His rightful place there. Jesus knew this would happen and told His disciples that He wouldn't always be with them. But He also made it quite clear that they would not be left alone: 'I will not leave you comfortless; I will come to you' (John 14:18). 'And I will pray the Father, and He will give you another Counsellor, (the Holy Spirit) to be with you for ever' (John 14:16).

We are reminded in Hebrews (13:5) that He has said: 'I will never leave you nor forsake you.' What wonderful promises to hold fast to when we feel alone and deserted. However, we need to claim them and make them our own. We have to seek after God and He will make His presence known and we will be able to rejoice in it. 'Let the hearts of those who seek the Lord rejoice! Seek the Lord and his strength, seek His presence continually!' (Psalm 105:3,4).

We know from experience that this is so true. God doesn't always remove the difficulties which make for loneliness and isolation. There have been long periods when I have been so ill that we have both been almost totally cut off from the outside world. Not only could we not get out but neither could we have people come to us. Any noise or exertion in the house on anyone's part, not just on mine, left me completely whacked!

At these times one is almost completely reliant on God for His companionship, love and care and He has never disappointed us or let us down. These have been times when prayer and reading the Bible have been almost impossible, let alone fellowship with others. Yet, I can honestly say that they have been most precious times of communing with God and totally satisfying. He has upheld me and I really haven't missed other people and activities. These have also been the times when I have felt God's presence most keenly and grown the most as a Christian.

When the situation has eased and we have a little more freedom I find I move on with renewed vigour and strength (even though my body may have taken a downward turn) and I am increasingly aware of God's closeness and presence. Formal prayer times and reading the Bible out of duty seem to be a thing of the past and we just 'commune' all day long. His friendship has become a most precious thing and something to be counted and treasured above all else.

2. Friends and family can be a great source of comfort

When God blesses us, He blesses us richly. Knowing Him might be the first and most important requisite but He doesn't intend for us to be always alone and apart from the rest of humanity. Going right back to creation God recognised that it was not good for man to be alone and created a helper and companion for him. In the same way he gives us family and friends and relationships without which we find it very hard to find true happiness. Yes, He can and does sustain completely and provide us with all we need but how good that He provides us with these other things too.

We have been so blessed with our family and circle of friends. They have been marvellous. Of course they have not always understood our situation and needs completely. Even when we try to explain in detail it's almost impossible to understand unless you've been in the same boat. And so sometimes their provision has fallen short. But we have seen the love and sincerity behind the actions and this has really lifted us and made us feel loved and cared for.

It must be really hard when friends and family desert one, but even if this happens alternative and new links can be established with other people. Susan may have been left high and dry by those she cared for most but she has learned to put that behind her. She is making other contacts. She found a life-line in her local carers support group. Now, much stronger, she is forming another group and reaching out to help others. This leads in to the third point.

3. Self help

Like Susan, we can help ourselves. Sometimes it can be hard and require a bit of effort but it is more than worth it. If we allow God into this situation too, He will more than help us to change and adapt and discover that life doesn't have to be lived in total isolation.

I am extremely handicapped and this does limit us very severely in many ways and yet I can truly say that loneliness and isolation are two things which we have overcome. How has it happened in a practical way?

Keep each other company
I do feel that a good relationship between carer and dependant, wherever possible, must make a big difference and co-operation seems to be the key word once again. I am only too aware how blessed we are in this and certainly do not take it for granted. Just as normal family relationships vary considerably, so it is between carer and dependant, and I realise that sometimes it is impossible, especially when the dependant is able to

respond very little or is perhaps unwilling to do so. However, many relationships can be improved with co-operation.

We have managed to remain good friends and try to put each other first. During the bad patches we are obviously together most of the time with little break, but we can choose to enjoy each other's company however limited we may be. It's good to have each other! At times this has meant talking about and sharing our happy memories, listening to music and cassettes or watching television or the birds in our garden. They are just simple pleasures but have prevented us from feeling alone at such times.

Maintain links with the outside world
When things have been a little improved, but we have still been fairly housebound, we have tried to maintain links with the outside world. Television, radio and newspapers can keep open the wider links, and letters and the telephone or even cassettes can keep us in touch with those things more personal and dear to us.

It is important not to give in to the temptation of shutting these out, feeling we have enough to cope with without bothering with all of this. We must not become small-minded and insular ... for our own good as much as anyone else's. The hardest people to relate to are those with no outlook or interest beyond their own and then perhaps they wonder why no one calls or writes. Some people, who are really old or handicapped or housebound, for whatever reason, can be like a 'breath of fresh air' because they have kept lively and alert to all that is happening around them even if they can't participate. Others, who probably have far less to bear, can become boring, cantankerous, grumbling, bitter and thoroughly miserable, and much is of their own making!

One thing which greatly helped us, during a period of being very housebound, was when one of the elders from our church came round and suggested that we might like to take over the weekly newssheet. It was suggested that people would be able to phone their notices through to us (as we were always in) and Chris could write them out and they could then be duplicated. We agreed, not knowing where we'd find the strength or energy or the incentive as we felt so out of touch with the life of the church.

But it was a wonderful idea and I'm sure God-given to prevent us from withdrawing further into our enforced isolation. We remained physically isolated for some time as I continued to be very ill. The effort involved in getting the newssheet together often felt too much. But we persevered and began to feel part of the fellowship again because, perhaps more than anyone, we knew exactly what was going on and were able to feel as if we had taken part in things and could certainly pray for them. People called for a reason, not just to ask after me or to give us some flowers. These things are lovely but when one has been cut off from life outside for months it's even nicer to feel useful and necessary again and not just someone who needs visiting!

Keep an open house
When things improved even further we tried to make our house an open one. Obviously we have severe limitations and cannot overdo anything but our home has become a useful one for holding meetings in. If I am in bed it doesn't matter at all, and Chris is able to join in with housegroups and prayer meetings and other church activities in the evening. The church has been very good about recognising this and is really willing to hold meetings in our house, if at all possible, to enable him to participate.

The church is our main 'activity' but this principle could equally apply to secular interests too. Indeed, as already mentioned when discussing the need for breaks, I stated that my husband invites friends in on a purely social basis and sometimes to share in his model railway hobby.

We have also tried to ensure an open home during the daytime and to encourage people to call - not just to 'visit the sick' - but as friends who we can have a two-way relationship with.

Indeed, there was a time when we felt in need of such fellowship. We had meetings but probably had to miss out on much of the social side of things. We decided to start an 'open house'. Every fortnight we opened our home for a two-hour period over lunchtime. We provided a simple ploughman's lunch and encouraged people to pop in even if only for half an hour. It worked really well. All sorts of people came; Mums with toddlers, old people, lonely people, people new to the area, those at work on a lunch-break and the unemployed. We had men as well as women which was lovely for Chris. Everyone came on the understanding that they would have to fend for themselves and that we could not wait on them. Having said that, it was still hard work and meant a whole day of preparation and clearing up afterwards for Chris, on top of the 'daily round'. It often exhausted me too but it was a lovely way of bringing people to us to fulfil our need, and I think it fulfilled a need in them too! It was eventually abandoned as we were asked to have a daytime study group in our home for those who, like us, find evenings difficult. We need to be flexible but we are certainly not lonely!

Some people, I know, do not feel they can do this and have deliberately cut themselves off from friends and outside contacts. Many feel it is too difficult and too much of an effort to bother with. Indeed my husband doesn't want too many evening activities - he is too busy and gets too tired and needs to relax on his own sometimes. But it is good to try and strike a balance between these two things.

Others feel that people cannot possibly be interested in them or want to be with them. They are so involved in an existence which is totally foreign to most people and it is hard to relate to normal everyday life or feel that other people want to relate to them. We are different and it is difficult but it is important for our own well-being to reach out to others. Mostly, we will be pleasantly surprised to discover that people do care about us and if we care about them too we can have a happy and worthwhile relationship, meeting each other's needs. For the carer's part this will prevent loneliness and help to keep a healthy perspective on life, thus avoiding introversion and withdrawal.

It can be embarrassing to have people in your home if the dependant is awkward and behaves strangely and again we can feel people won't want to come. But it is still worth being open and trying. Tell people what your situation is like and they can choose. You may lose some friends but true friends will stick by you and still want to come because of you!

Try to go out and mix with others
When possible, we do try to get out and mix with people. As already mentioned, breaks are vital for the carer on his own. But there are things we can do together if at all possible. It's good to meet with like-minded people and there are voluntary groups springing up not only for the carer but for those concerned with the handicap of the dependant, whether physical, mental or just relating to age. (This will be dealt with more fully in chapter 13.)

It's also good to mix with ordinary people. This will usually mean being prepared to adapt but ways can usually be found round problems. Some buildings are not suitable for wheelchairs and so for us this means we cannot go to everything we would like. Neither can we stay too long as not only do I get too tired but there is always the problem of the loo! We are so fortunate in that our Sunday morning service takes place in a suitable building. When we can't attend evening activities we always look for suitable daytime alternatives and so far have found them. This means our days, which are short anyway, get an awful lot packed into them and we have to be sensible and learn when to stop.

Thora's story is an encouraging account of how one can step out sometimes if one is willing to. She recounts how she and her husband went to Australia to visit their daughter and family. At first, when they were asked, it seemed out of the question. Her husband, Bill, is severely disabled with arthritis. He is wheelchair-bound, in a lot of pain, on a lot of medication and needs frequent dressings and nursing care for a chronic infection in his knee. But they made enquiries. They decided to take the risk and went for five months. They found plenty of help available on the journey and when they were over there. The health care was good and they had no problems. They saw all sorts of places, did lots of things and had a wonderful time. Thora sums it all up by saying: 'We have many happy memories and photos to remind us of a holiday we thought would be impossible for us to undertake.'

Circumstances may vary considerably for individuals and never stay the same but we are learning to accept them and to adapt and explore every possibility to make life as full as possible during each particular phase of our lives. It is not easy, requiring much effort and willingness to adapt and also allowing others to share in our needs, but in so doing we both live very full lives and seldom have a moment to feel lonely, even in the darkest patches.

Chapter 11
THE BEREAVED CARER

'However hard today is, there will come a day when it was not for long enough': so Ruth had to keep reminding herself as she cared for her dying father. Many carers are looking after someone who is elderly or very ill or perhaps both. At some point they will be bereaved.

However hard it has been for them, most have cared out of love rather than duty. For many it has been an enjoyable experience. John, who cared for his senile mother for 22 years says: 'I don't regret one day of those years. In a curious way I enjoyed them, despite the fact I had a business to run.'

Other carers have found it a very rewarding experience. Amy cared for her elderly, failing mother when she came to live with her and her husband. 'I treasured those years,' she says, 'and learned much from Mother's wisdom.'

Many speak of learning a great deal from the one they care for. Sarah, who is still in the process of caring for her mentally and physically handicapped sister, says, 'She has taught me so much. She hears the birds singing in an aviary, talks to cats and dogs and feels pity for a man walking along using two sticks. With such a person as my sister in the house one is constantly brought up to appreciate how good life is.'

With such positive thoughts it is hardly surprising that most carers will experience all the usual feelings of grief, sorrow and loss. They have all had difficult times but most will be able to echo the sentiment of Linda (who had a particularly hard relationship with her mother) when she says: 'I still miss her a lot.'

The grieving period has already been explored, in detail, when looking at the losses experienced by the carer. There is really very little to add about this normal process except to repeat that it is just as important, when an actual death has occurred, to take time to mourn and not to suppress one's feelings. There are books on the market better able than I am to help a bereaved person come to terms with their loss.

However, it is worth mentioning two aspects which, although not exclusive to a carer, are perhaps more likely to be experienced by them than other bereaved people.

1. Relief

However much one misses the person who has died there is often a sense of relief. Relief for oneself because it has been a strain as well as a joy. But mainly relief for the loved one. As Linda says: 'I must admit I felt a sense of relief when she died ... at knowing she was safe in the Lord's hands and freed from the frustrations of her handicap.' It is always hard to watch a loved one suffer and such sentiments are quite natural and normal.

2. Guilt

This is perhaps a more serious problem and also very prevalent. As such it needs looking at in greater depth.

Many carers feel they haven't done their best. As we've already seen, guilt occurs often when the dependant is still being cared for. But if it is not dealt with at the time or perhaps if the person has been completely bowled over by the circumstances surrounding their caring role (particularly if it is a short, action packed period with little time to think straight and adapt), guilt and remorse can quickly set in after the death of the loved one.

For those who have a fairly smooth, lengthy period of caring it seems to get dealt with along the way and when the death of the loved one eventually happens, guilt does not seem to be such a problem to deal with.

But if it has been a tumultuous time, whether for a long or short period, then the carer is more likely to feel they have failed and feel very guilty about it. Even if the shortcomings are very minor in other people's eyes, to the already grieving carer they can grow out of all proportion. It appears that they seldom got anything right and as it's too late to do anything about it now they revert to 'if onlys': 'If only I'd done so and so.' 'If only I had been more patient.' 'If only I'd spent more time with her.' And so it continues!

Jackie and her husband cared for his Gran because they wanted to make her last years happy. She was only with them for three years and she was happy and contented for most of the time. But the pressures began to mount. They had two small children and friction built up between Jackie's husband and his Gran. He would get angry about the extra work she caused and Gran would get upset. She would argue with him and boss him about which made him feel resentful. Jackie had to be a peacemaker. When Gran died, Jackie's husband took a long time to recover from his guilt at being resentful.

Pam was separated from her husband with a three year-old son when her mother was diagnosed as having cancer. Pam was a fully trained nurse and didn't think twice about having her mother come to stay with them as her condition worsened.

But caring for her mother was different from caring for her hospital patients. She often felt as if she were getting it all wrong. As her Mum neared the end of her life things got more difficult for Pam. She discovered that her husband had been sexually abusing their son on his access visits. Her son needed her. She had to cope with police officers and health visitors as her mother lay dying in the room next door. Small wonder she didn't know which way to turn or what should take priority!

The morning her mother died she could take no more. She was sleeping in the sitting room with her mother. When she awoke, hearing her mother's laboured, heavy breathing, she knew the end was very near. She kissed her mother and left the room to get washed and dressed because she couldn't face being with her mother when she died. After about ten minutes, when it was obvious her mother had stopped breathing, she returned to do all the necessary things and phone the doctor. Pam has since gone through a lot of guilt and remorse, especially concerning the very last moments of her mother's life.

How can one cope with these feelings of guilt?

Recognise that everyone fails
We are human beings. We are not perfect. We all fall short of God's perfect standard. We will all fail sometimes particularly under stress. We are all selfish, resentful, angry, impatient and unloving at times. Romans 7:19 puts it thus: 'For I do not do the good I want, but the evil I do not want is what I do.'

Recognise we don't have to bear the blame
It is so easy to get completely weighed down with our failings. Paul speaks for everyone when he says 'Wretched man that I am! Who will deliver me from this body of death?' (Romans 7:24).

But, fortunately for us, we needn't remain in despair. Paul didn't. He knew there was a solution. It was (and still is) found through Jesus Christ (Romans 7:25). Because of what Jesus did for us, because He died for us on the cross and took the punishment for all our wrongdoings and failings, we need not bear our shame and guilt. He bears it for us. We can be delivered from our predicament.

How

All we have to do is to respond to God. We do this by recognising and acknowledging that we do fail (or sin) but that Jesus Christ has died for us and taken our guilt away.

We then ask God to forgive us for our sins and *believe* that he has done so. I want to emphasise the 'believe' part because this is where so many people come unstuck. They keep on asking for forgiveness. Not necessary! When we ask for forgiveness, God forgives and forgets. There is no point in keeping on asking because God doesn't know what we're talking about. Our fault or failure has been forgotten about as soon as we bring it to Him. 'As far as the east is from the west, so far does He remove our transgressions from us.' (Psalm 103:12). What a comforting thought and if we can only grasp it, not just with our minds but also allow it to sink into our hearts, our guilt will vanish and our peace return.

Once forgiven we don't have to keep struggling for protection

If we also ask Jesus Christ to take control of our lives, God's Spirit will come and dwell inside us, enabling us to triumph over our weaknesses and faults. He can change us and make us more like Jesus. But it won't all happen overnight. It's a process that takes a lifetime and we will still fail ... even as Christians. We will fail every time we try and take back that control. But that doesn't matter as long as we are ready to confess to God that we have failed and allow His forgiveness to operate once more.

We no longer need feel guilty

If only we accept this we no longer need to feel condemned and guilty. Paul says: 'There is therefore now no condemnation for those who are in Christ Jesus' (Romans 8:1). We have been justified by our faith in Christ (Romans 5:1) and through His blood shed for us (Romans 5:9). To be justified is to be treated by God as righteous or as the best definition has it 'just as if we had never sinned'

For those who are already Christians and say, 'I know all that but I still feel guilty', my answer is: 'Don't rely on your feelings.' Feel guilty all you like but that doesn't alter the fact that you are no longer guilty in God's eyes (if you have asked His forgiveness through Jesus Christ). If you don't feel forgiven then keep repeating some of these wonderful assurances, from the book of Romans, which I have been quoting. Before long you will discover that you 'feel' forgiven too, for God's word does not lie and He will make it real to you.

There is one more thing to be said about guilt. All the above applies if we are actually guilty of failing in some way. But some bereaved carers will conjure up feelings of guilt which are totally unfounded. It's no good asking for forgiveness if there is nothing to forgive. How do you know whether your guilt is reasonable or not?

* Ask God to show you. He will. If you continue to be genuinely bothered about something perhaps you do need to ask forgiveness. But if you keep having dragged to your minds things which you know God has dealt with and if you continue to feel condemned and wretched, this is not from God and there is no need for guilt to persist. Believe what God says.

* Take notice of what friends and relatives tell you. If they say you have nothing to feel guilty about and that you've done your best and what you knew was right, then they are probably right. They can see things more objectively than someone in a bereaved state. Even if you can't accept their assurances immediately, hold on to them until they make sense.

* Believe your own common sense. Perhaps not immediately, because you may not be able to think or behave rationally, but eventually try to look back. Try to be objective. Try to get things into perspective. Did you do your best? Was your loved one basically happy and grateful? If they weren't, why not? Was it your fault or was it because they were difficult by nature, or frightened or in pain? Even if it wasn't perfect were conditions the best they could be under the circumstances?

Pam, despite the guilt and remorse, can look back and see that even though she failed sometimes, her mother 'Had a lot more love and care than she would ever have done except in a hospice and there,' she admits, 'the home environment would have been missing. Above all, I feel secure in knowing that I did my best. Maybe it is less than I thought it should be but I know that if I was in the same position and my son was unable to cope, I would never blame him, because he's my son and I love him. If my Mum had known then I'm sure this would have been her attitude too.'

There really is no more to say except to summarise it all by saying that if one has a right relationship with God, one will also be made right with oneself and with others and the guilt will vanish. As Pam puts it, the 'shoulds' and 'oughts' and 'wish I hads' only last a little while. The good memories - joy, laughter and happiness - stay forever.

Chapter 12
HOW TO RECEIVE HELP —
FROM THE STATE

Having identified and explored many of the problem areas for the carer, both those within our own experience and those that are the experiences of others with whom we have come into contact, I would like to stress that such areas need to be overcome and dealt with personally. However much help is available from other sources it can never really be used on its own to deal with personal issues which need to be faced. If we treat it as such and expect it to be the answer to all our problems we will be disappointed. It can become a scapegoat, and we may well blame the system or other Christians or the church or anything else for that matter. It is so much easier to put the blame elsewhere, especially when we are vulnerable and hurting, rather than face up to putting right that which is wrong within ourselves.

No system is perfect; they are often inadequate. People like Chris and me are in a good position now (after 15 years experience) to point out and try and change some of the bad things (and this we try and do in our own small ways). But we do not do so out of anger or when our wounds are still raw. Having overcome many of the initial problems, we are able to do so rationally and almost objectively, with a view to making life that bit easier for those who come after us.

For instance, we waited over 18 months to get important alterations done to our house. In fact, after more than two years they still had not been completed. The 'system' takes time even in 'priority cases' like ours. When you are denied the basic things which everyone else takes for granted (like using the toilet, having a bath and being able to get outside one's house unaided in an emergency) it would be easy to get irate, but funnily enough we no longer do. Such things, important as they are, have been put into perspective. I have discovered other carers often have the same outlook. It can be frustrating, annoying and makes life that bit more difficult - and of course we try our hardest to get things put right - but it is not a major disaster compared with what we have already gone through.

So, although there is much help available which can ease the strain enormously, it will never be perfect in this imperfect world and should be looked at accordingly. But perhaps it is now time to look, in more detail, at the kind of help available ... practical and personal. Let's start with statutory help.

Wherever you live there are statutory services which, in theory, should be able to meet many of your needs. Indeed it is the right of a disabled person or his carer to receive an assessment of their needs, by the local authority, according to The Disabled Persons (Services, Consultation and Representation) Act, 1986.

However, the services will not as a general rule come to you and so it is important to not only know what is available but also where to find it! It must also be stressed that facilities will vary from area to area. The service you need may just not be available or is so overstretched that there is either a long waiting list or have people with a higher priority who come first.

Generally, health services are the concern of the district health authority (or district health board in Scotland), social services and education come under the control of the county council, and housing under the control of the district council. Certain services are provided jointly between them.

The whole system is really rather complex, but one way to simplify it is to concentrate on the two (possibly three) key figures who can open the doors to almost everything else.

GP (General Practitioner). It is important for carer as well as dependant to receive all the medical care possible and obviously your GP will treat you accordingly. A good GP should also provide you with advice, information and support and can be the opening to many other medical services.

He can organise for you:

A District Nurse who can help with the practical jobs of caring for someone at home. They can come on a regular basis or just occasionally when a need arises. They can help with dressings, injections, bathing, toileting, lifting and turning. They will also advise on such areas as incontinence and bed sores and possibly arrange for suitable equipment (like incontinence aids, hoists, special bed or mattress, bed rails or bath seat and commode) and people to help you (like a night nurse or auxiliary nurse).

A **Health Visitor** who can listen to your day-to-day worries and suggest practical ways of coping. They can also tell you about your local services, help you make contact with them and help you arrange for any home adaptations or aids that you may need. However, in many areas they are usually so busy dealing with young children that they have little time to spare for the disabled or carers.

An **Occupational Therapist**. This service can be provided by the social services or the health authority. A community O.T. employed by the health authority and based in a hospital will have out patient referrals as well as in patient ones but this will more often be done by the hospital specialist than the GP.

A **Physiotherapist** who can visit people who have difficulty with mobility in their own home and offer treatment and advice on how to keep as mobile and fit as possible. They provide various kinds of therapy to suit the need. They can also advise the carer on the simplest and best ways to lift and move the dependant without hurting himself. However, this service is only rarely a domiciliary one. Transport can be provided to the hospital instead. It is also more likely to be the responsibility of the hospital specialist rather than the GP.

A **Community Psychiatric Nurse** deals with people who have mental problems visiting them at home. They not only keep an eye on the patient and carer but can also give medication or refer the person back to their GP or specialist if necessary. Their support and experience can be invaluable for a carer dealing with someone who behaves difficulty.

A **Speech Therapist** who can help language disorders arising from handicap, illness or injury. They are usually based at schools or clinics but can sometimes visit a person at home.

A **Chiropodist** who can help people to stay as mobile as possible through proper foot care. They are provided under the NHS to OAPs, both the mentally and physically handicapped and children under 16, and can be found in hospital or health centre clinics. Transport can be provided for such visits if necessary or the person can sometimes be visited in the home.

A **Continence Adviser** is also available in some areas to assess and treat the problem (if possible) and to offer advice on how to deal with it. Often the district nurse can put you in touch with a continence adviser rather than the GP doing so.

The GP can also:

* refer your dependant to a hospital for more specialised treatment.

* arrange for an assessment at a child development centre if there is one. They are usually attached to your local hospital and many professionals are involved (e.g. paediatricians, speech therapists, physiotherapists, specialist health visitors, teachers, social workers and occupational thera-pists).

* arrange for admission to a hospital or home for a short period to enable the carer to take a short break or holiday (respite care), or in the case of an emergency.

* refer you (in some areas) to a district handicap team, district disability team or district mental handicap team. Such teams include professional people from both the health and social services and sometimes a repre-sentative from a local voluntary organisation. They can pool their knowl-edge and co-operate in providing the best facilities for individuals.

* help provide a wheelchair, although a visit to the nearest Disabled Service Centre is usually necessary in order to be assessed properly. These are usually rather few and far between and in some areas 'out clinics' known as Wheelchair Assessment Centres are being set up in designated hospitals. This means one may not have to travel quite so far for a wheelchair assessment. The GP can provide some other medical aids too.

* also help you in trying to get the following: a home carer, care attendant, some state allowances, council housing, meals on wheels, laundry service, a review of benefits, day care, residential care and sheltered accommodation.

Social Worker. A social worker is able to help in a number of ways dealing with personal, financial and practical issues. It is the duty of a social worker to inform you of local authority services but he often knows quite a lot about local voluntary services too. He can be contacted at your local social services department which will be found in the phone book under your local county council authority. You can either arrange an appointment at their office or for a home visit.

Your social worker should be able to organise:

An Occupational Therapist (who is often employed by the local authority and based in the social services department). They will visit the disabled person in his own home and teach him and his carer to manage everyday tasks and to suggest aids and equipment which might further enable them to cope. There are all sorts of non-medical aids available for help with hygiene, dressing, feeding and household tasks as well as special chairs, wheelchair or buggy and play equipment and sometimes alarm systems. Much of the equipment can be loaned. They can advise on adaptations to the home like altering or installing a bathroom downstairs, providing ramps for access, and fitting a stair lift etc. On their recommen-dation to the local environmental health department you may be able to receive a grant. If you live in a council house the adaptations will usually be paid for by the local authority. Otherwise you may be able to receive quite a substantial grant but it will involve a means test to establish the amount you qualify for.

A Home Carer who used to be called a home-help and who could help with cleaning the house. Due to demand and financial restrictions this service is usually no longer available. Instead, their main role is caring - assisting people to get up in the morning, assisting with dressing, providing meals, lighting fires, shopping and assisting the person to bed at night. In theory they not only help people living on their own but also a carer if he is unable to manage unaided and as such they can be a valuable help. However, the demand for home carers is so great that in some areas they can only be provided for the elderly or disabled who live alone. Most local authorities will charge for a home carer and the amount will depend on your financial circumstances. (They can also be obtained by contacting your social services department direct without going through your social worker).

A Care Attendant who can provide various kinds of help depending on your need. Such help could include jobs around the house and also help with washing and dressing, help to enable you both get out together or sitting with the person you care for while you take a break. The hours are flexible too and in some schemes can even include night assistance. As with the home carer there is usually a small charge for the service.

A Sitting or Minding Service which can give you either a regular or occasional break. Most sitters are not specially trained but will often have experience in caring. Some will be able to do the jobs a carer has to do - either around the house or for the dependant - while others will just provide companionship and keep an eye on the person you care for.

Meals on Wheels are for those who are unable to cook themselves a meal. They provide a hot midday meal on several days a week and in some areas at weekends too. If you are at work during the day or care for someone not in your household they can be supplied for the person you are looking after.

A Laundry Service which is usually for bed linen, for people with incontinence, but other items can be included. There is usually a small charge.

NB. All the above services can be bought privately but are very expensive. However, if your local authority or local voluntary groups are inadequate they may be worth considering.

The social worker can also organise:

Facilities for Young Children including a place at a play centre, nursery or play group.

A Day Centre or Sheltered Workshop including facilities very similar to those provided by a day hospital

Respite Care which provides short-term residential care or fostering to give you a break or in an emergency.

Holidays for your dependant alone or with you as well.

Residential Care either on a permanent basis if you can no longer cope or on a shared basis enabling your dependant to come home for weekends, visits or perhaps for a week or two every month. The fees for all of these will vary considerably depending on your need and circumstances.

Hospital Specialist or Consultant. The person you care for may have been referred to a hospital specialist by his GP and be being treated for his condition either in hospital or an out patients department. (If it is very difficult to get to the hospital appointment, your GP can arrange for the specialist to see your dependant at home). Such specialists often understand the problems involved in caring for a sick, handicapped or elderly person and it is worth discussing any difficulties with them. They can organise many of the services that a GP can and also:

A Day Hospital Place which provides training, treatment and social activities for the dependant and enables the carer to have a break or be employed.

A Short Stay in Hospital either for treatment or respite care.

Regular Short Stays in Hospital

Permanent Care in Hospital

Physiotherapy in the hospital as an outpatient and which might include treatment in a hydro-therapy pool or possibly (but not very likely) physiotherapy treatment at home

Referral to an Occupational Therapist employed by the health authority.

Referral to the Appliance Department of the hospital to be fitted and supplied with things like splints, special footwear, corsets etc.

Referral to the Disabled Service Centre to be assessed and fitted for things like artificial limbs and wheelchairs (or to the wheelchair assessment centre if there is one).

Although these three key figures can put you in touch with almost every service you may require there are one or two other places to mention:

Education comes under the management of the local county council who by law are required to provide free education for any child with special needs up to the age of 16 and are obliged to assess any child over two (or under two at the parent's request) whom they think may have special needs. Many professional people (teachers, educational psychologist, GP, specialist, social worker etc.) will be involved in making the assessment and in recommending how such needs should be met. This will be reviewed annually, but if you have any worries or queries ask to speak to the educational adviser for children with special needs, at your local education authority.

Portage is a national charity which has been incorporated into the local education authority and receives full funding from them. It is a home based programme for the carer/parents of a pre school child with special needs. It aims to teach the skills which will enable the parents to cope with their child and his needs and to encourage them to help him to reach his full potential. It gives the carer a structure to work within - perhaps with a daily teaching session for parent and child to follow. It encourages the carer to feel that his role is vitally important and very worthwhile. It also provides much needed support and counsel, particularly when parents are still coming to terms with the grief surrounding the knowledge that their child is handicapped in some way. General advice on such things as what benefits they may be entitled to receive and liaison with other professionals who may be needed, like physiotherapists and speech therapists, is also an important part of the work. It usually involves a weekly visit to the home of the carer and child. A doctor or hospital specialist can refer a parent or carer to this service or it can be sought by the parents themselves.

The Housing Department (under your local district council) can offer advice on council homes, sheltered accommodation and local housing schemes.

The Citizens Advice Bureau or local advice centre can offer all sorts of general advice dealing with benefits, rights, legal matters, education and housing. We have found the Citizens Advice Bureau to be really helpful and if they don't know all the answers on the day you phone, they will often make an appointment for you to see someone else, another day, who is more knowledgeable in the area you are seeking advice about.

D.S.S. for all government benefits and financial help. Caring for someone costs money and it is important to find out about all the benefits which are available to you both and to sort your finances out. This can be really complicated. There are many government benefits available but there are four main ones for the carer and his dependant to consider:

Attendance Allowance is paid to people who need a lot of looking after because they are severely mentally or physically disabled (i.e. looking after with regard to their bodily functions or because they are a danger to themselves or others and need constant supervision. It does not mean help with household tasks). It can be paid to people of any age. There are two rates: the lower rate is for daytime attendance, the higher rate for night attendance as well. It is tax-free and can normally be paid in full on top of any other Social Security benefits. A medical assessment will be necessary in order to be awarded it.

Mobility Allowance can be claimed for those who are between the ages of 5 and 65 who are unable, or virtually unable, to walk. It can be paid until a person is 80 as long as they qualified for it before they reached the age of 65. It too is tax-free and will not be affected by any other benefits. It will also usually need a medical assessment.

Invalid Care Allowance is a weekly benefit for carers who spend at least 35 hours a week looking after someone who qualifies for Attendance Allowance or Constant Attendance Allowance. You can claim if you are aged between 16 and 60 (for a woman) or 16 and 65 (for a man). It is not means tested but it is taxable and may well affect other benefits you are receiving.

Severe Disablement Allowance for those who are too sick or disabled for work but can't get Sickness Benefit or Invalidity Benefit because they haven't paid enough NI contributions. (If you have paid enough contributions and become sick or disabled whilst working you would normally get Sickness Benefit for 6 months and then qualify for Invalidity Benefit). You can apply for S.D.A. if you are of working age and haven't been able to work for at least six months.

NB. The government have recently issued a document called 'The Way Ahead' which sets out changes which are likely to be made, over the next year or two, with regard to benefits concerning the disabled. Some of these have already started to be set in motion (e.g. S.D.A. in Dec. 1990 will receive an age-related addition - the rate being dependent on one's age when one became incapacitated. The earnings related addition to Invalidity Benefit is being phased out from April 1991). There are also proposals for new benefits in 1992 - one of which is a new Disability Allowance. This is basically the merging of Attendance Allowance and Mobility Allowance with different rates depending on the severity of one's disability).

Apart from the above benefits, if you are unable to work because you are caring for someone, there is financial help available which since April 1988 has been known as **Income Support**. This is money on which to live, but it will be means tested. For instance, it is reduced by the amount of Severe Disablement Allowance or Invalid Care Allowance you receive, savings over £3,000, and some other forms of income. However, it does take into account special needs, e.g. there are premiums for carers and disabled people. If you are buying your own home you may be able to get help with your mortgage interest as part of your Income Support.

The benefit system really is very complex. Any advice will initially only be very general and may appear confusing and conflicting. If in doubt just keep asking!

For instance, they will often tell you to claim for benefits because there are long term advantages irrespective of whether you receive any extra money. The other 'long term advantages' are not made clear, but we have discovered after a lot of enquiry that they are mostly to do with getting National Insurance credits which enable you to protect your retirement pension and your sickness benefit entitlements. This seems a very important consideration, but it is not stressed, and one often doesn't bother to claim benefits one is entitled to when one will not actually receive more money.

However, Invalid Care Allowance is taxable and so it might not always be advantageous to claim it. If in doubt contact your local Tax Office. The address is in the phone book under 'Inland Revenue'.

If you cannot get Invalid Care Allowance but are looking after someone who gets Attendance Allowance or Constant Attendance Allowance, the Home Responsibilities Protection scheme can help to protect your right to basic Retirement Pension (although not sickness benefit). Contact your local D.S.S.

If you are in receipt of certain state benefits or on a low income, there are many extra benefits you may be entitled to, such as: **Housing Benefit** (an allowance to help pay your rent); **Community Charge Benefit** (an allowance to help you with your Community Charge); **N.H.S. Benefits** (free prescriptions, dental care, eye tests and vouchers for glasses, travelling costs to hospital etc.); **Help from the Social Services Dept.** for such things as fares, nurseries or playgroups, special equipment, home adaptations, holidays, home helps, residential accommodation, day centres, meals on wheels, special housing, laundry and provision of television or telephone.

There is also a *social fund* for people who face a sudden or exceptional expense which they cannot immediately pay for out of regular income. Some payments are grants - e.g. to help a disabled or elderly person lead an independent life in the community. But most are loans - e.g. to help pay for essential items of furniture, repairs, household equipment, travel costs etc. There are also payments available during exceptionally cold weather or to help with funeral expenses.

If you wish to obtain more information about any of these benefits ask at your local Social Security office. There is also a free advice service (tel.

0800 666 555) which is very helpful and can often provide more detailed information than your local office. Again, the Citizens Advice Bureau is a very helpful place to contact; or ask at your library for *The Disability Rights Handbook* (Disability Alliance) which offers a very complete guide to the rights and benefits available to a disabled person and which is updated every April.

As I have already said, the whole system is very complicated, often inadequate and always overstretched. We still don't understand it all after many years of using it and, of course, just when you think you've got it sorted out - it all changes! But please don't give up. It can supply you with the valuable practical and financial help and advice that you will need in order to both lead as full and as comfortable a life as possible.

Chapter 13
HOW TO RECEIVE HELP —
FROM VOLUNTARY GROUPS
AND SCHEMES

There is a large variety of voluntary groups and community schemes offering practical help and support to all kinds of people ... carer included. They can often bridge any gaps in the statutory services and are well worth investigating.

They are nonprofit-making and largely rely on donations to fund them ,although some receive financial support from local authorities or the government.

Some groups are national whereas others operate only locally. The services and facilities available will vary greatly depending on where you live and although I can give a general outline of the kind of help which could be available, it is important to check within your own locality what provision there is.

There is a variety of ways of finding out what is available. Before you make enquiries though, it is probably advisable to decide on what sort of help you require, rather than ask in general terms about what is available. When you have decided, here are some suggestions of who to contact:

Your **social worker, GP, health visitor, district nurse** or **hospital specialist.**

A central office in your area which may be called (depending on where you live) a **Council for Voluntary Service, Voluntary Service Council, Voluntary Action Group** or a **Rural Community Council**. Look in the telephone directory or in the Yellow Pages under 'Charitable and benevolent organisations'. If you have any difficulty, try writing to: (for England) National Council for Voluntary Organisations, 26 Bedford Square, London WC1B 3HU or (for Wales) Wales Council for Voluntary Action, Crescent Rd, Caerphilly, Mid Glamorgan CF8 1XL.

Citizens Advice Bureau or local advice centre.

Public library.
Town Hall Information Office.
A local volunteer bureau which can advise you about individual volunteers. Look in the telephone directory under **Volunteer Bureau, Volunteer Centre, Voluntary Work Centre** or **Voluntary Workers Bureau.** Or you can contact the **Volunteer Centre Information Department,** 29 Lower King's Rd, Berkhamstead, Herts HP4 2AB.

Look under **Disabled - amenities and information** in your local Yellow Pages.

DIAL, which stands for Disablement Information and Advice Line (some areas only), can be found in the Yellow Pages under 'Disabled'.

Voluntary schemes and groups should be able to provide all sorts of practical or advisory help. Different groups will offer different services and you will obviously not need or be drawn to all of them. However, I have tried to summarise some of the main ones which could be helpful to a carer.

Groups concerned with the same illness or disability

There are far too many organisations to mention in this category! It would not be an exaggeration to say that just about every illness or disability is catered for ... ranging from the very rare, to such common things as cancer and arthritis. Many of them produce useful publications and newsletters as well as providing other services. They often have local groups where you and your dependant can meet with people in similar circumstances. As well as being able to let off steam and talk to people who understand because they've had similar experiences, it is also a good place to swap information and ideas on how to cope. Many of these groups organise their own self-help schemes and information. Sometimes they become involved in campaigning for better facilities locally as well as fund-raising. Often they meet a social need with outings and suitable activities. If you wish to find out if there is an organisation suited to your needs, ask at your local library. They may have a book called the *Voluntary Agencies Directory* (National Council for Voluntary Organisations 1988) or from the list at the back of the *Disability Rights Handbook* (Disability Alliance - revised every year).

More general groups

Most specific illnesses or disabilities also come into a wider category like the elderly or the mentally handicapped, and it is worth contacting some of these more general groups. For example:
Age Concern
Help the Aged

Contact a Family (for children with special needs)
MIND (for mentally ill people)
MENCAP (for people with mental handicaps).

Carers Groups

There is a national group for carers called the **Carers National Association**. The address is: 29 Chilworth Mews, London W2 3RG. As with the other groups dealing with specific illnesses or disabilities, it can offer much help, support and advice.

There are also many carers groups being formed across the country. Some may be attached to the national group or run by other voluntary organisations or possibly run by the social services department. At such groups you will be able to meet and share with other carers. If you can't or don't want to attend the meetings they can often put you in touch with another carer in your area who you can share with. Many groups have volunteers who operate a sitting service for your dependant to enable you both to have a break from each other. Some groups can offer carers training in basic nursing skills, or in dealing with particular problems like incontinence or lifting.

Practical support and help for the carer are provided by **Crossroads Care**, 10 Regent Place, Rugby, Warwickshire CV21 2PN. The scheme operates in many areas throughout the country providing practical support and help, either on a regular basis, perhaps just one or two hours a week to enable them to have a break, or in an emergency if they fall ill. They have trained care attendants and their aims are to relieve stress and to allow disabled people the chance to carry on in their own homes if a breakdown in the household occurs. They seek to work alongside existing statutory services rather than replace them.

Barnardo's is a national organisation providing help and support to more than 16,000 needy young people and their families each year. One group they have always supported are those with a mental handicap. They have begun an Advocacy Service which can step in and ensure the youngster is provided for and their interests taken into account if, and when, the parents can no longer cope. In doing this it can take much of the pressure and anxiety from parents who worry about the future. It is a free service but it is only available to those families connected with Barnardo's already. It is funded entirely by voluntary donations and because of the numbers of people involved it is only able to operate in the North West and Scotland at the moment. But because of the demand, Barnado's are seeking ways to receive more funding and thus expand this work to other regions in the future.

Counselling

Much help, advice and counsel can be received from all the statutory and voluntary organisations already mentioned, but sometimes more specific counsel is needed on a more personal level which they may not be able to provide.

Professional counsellors are available. **The British Association for Counselling**, 37A Sheep Street, Rugby, Warwickshire CV21 3BX, can inform you of recommended counsellors in your area. The fees will vary. Some will charge according to your financial state and a few may be free.

Relate (formerly The National Marriage Guidance Council) has local branches where you can get help or counselling on sexual and marital problems. Look in the phone book under ' Relate Marriage Guidance'.

SPOD (Sexual and Personal Relationship of People with a Disability) provides similar information but specially intended for people with disabilities and related problems. The address is: 286 Camden Rd, London N7 0JB.

Family friends and neighbours

This is perhaps the most obvious sort of 'voluntary' support available to the carer! Not everyone can call on such people but many, many carers can testify (as we can) to the wonderful help that is so willingly and faithfully offered.

Chapter 14
WHAT HELP IS AVAILABLE FROM CHRISTIANS

It is true to say that of all the kinds of help we have explored so far some of it will come from Christians. Christian doctors, nurses, social workers etc. are all quite common. Many Christians get involved in voluntary work too and many of us will have Christian friends, neighbours and perhaps other members of our family living nearby.

This has certainly been our experience and has been a real blessing. They may not have always understood our position - perhaps not as much as some non-Christians who have had specific experience of carers and their needs - but it has been good to know that our outlook and spiritual reactions have been similar. They have added that extra dimension to things which, unfortunately, is sometimes missing from all the non-Christian help and support we have received (although this has been marvellous too).

I know it is true of the experience of many other carers too. Mary has found the support of her church invaluable especially in taking her husband out and giving her a break. 'The church has helped a lot ... it's nice when he goes out of an evening sometimes. It gives me a break and I can relax knowing he's being well cared for. I am free to be myself even if it only means sitting in a chair and doing nothing.'

Although I fully appreciate all the many Christians who do give so freely of their time in helping needy people and also those who are employed in the caring professions, I have been saddened and frustrated in writing and researching this book to discover that there are also many Christians and Christian organisations that are lagging sadly behind in their understanding and involvement with carers and their dependants. To so many the carer is still an unheard of and underestimated member of society and as such is being neglected by the Christian community. This is why I have had to put the statutory and voluntary help first ... because this is where most of the help and recognition is coming from!

Sarah cares for her sister Joy who is 49 years old and physically and mentally handicapped. Her 83 year-old mother has also recently come to live with them as she is no longer able to care for herself. Sarah and her husband were members of a caring church where she was very active and happy. But she and her husband moved some miles away just a month before Joy came to live with them.

It was assumed that because Sarah had always been very active for her church this would continue. She was asked to help with the Girl's Brigade, the Women's Work and a Housegroup. Nobody seemed to realise she had a sister to care for now and this was followed three years later by a mother too. Sarah says 'At no time was I asked if the church could help me. Truly I felt like screaming: "Don't ask me to help you, tell me what you can do to help me".'

Once, Sarah was asked to speak at a meeting. 'Can someone pick me up,' she asked. 'Joy can't get on and off a bus.'

'Can't you leave her at home?' was the reply.

Sarah stuck it out at the church hoping help would come her way. It didn't. Only one busy young mum could see that she needed a break. In the end she contacted a social worker who, she says, has been wonderful to her. She comments 'Sad to see how over-worked Social Services are compared to the church and how they care.'

Sarah's friend told her a story about a doctor who visited his vicar requesting help for a young mum whose husband was unwell. All she wanted was someone to meet a child from school. 'Sorry old boy,' the vicar said 'we don't have anyone living in that part of town ... hold on why don't we contact Social Services. I think I have their numbers here.' The doctor told Sarah's friend 'I was sad - sad to think no one in the church could have helped.' The doctor had, in fact, thought of Social Services first himself and had all the numbers in his surgery but he just thought maybe the church could help.

Hopefully, such incidents are not too frequent - I'm sure Sarah would be the first to agree that many churches are, of course, extremely caring towards their own members and extend this help to those outside whenever they see a need - but perhaps they occur frequently enough to give a word of reproach and challenge to some Christians not to be like this!

Indeed, I did find some encouraging pieces of information. I had to hunt quite hard for them and my discoveries may not be complete by any means but if there are any other specifically Christian organisations out there, involved with carers in any way, then I apologise for not including them!

I discovered two national organisations who are aware of the needs of carers and are beginning to investigate and meet their needs. The first is only concerned with caring for the elderly and whilst this is by far the largest group of people being cared for, it only further emphasises the lack of provision for carers in general.

* The first organisation is **The Christian Council on Ageing** (The Old Court, Greens Norton, Nr. Towcester, Northants NN12 8BS). It is a national voluntary organisation but wishes to develop at a local level. It is interdenominational and membership is open to 'any individual who professes faith in Jesus Christ'. It publishes a quarterly journal, runs courses and seminars, publishes occasional papers and encourages the setting-up of retired groups and counselling services for the elderly at a local level. It is not specifically concerned with informal care, being intended to make churches more aware of the potential of elderly people as well as seeing to their needs, but its aims include improving 'pastoral support and fellowship for those who care for elderly people.'

* The second is the **Jubilee Centre** (Jubilee House, 3 Hooper Street, Cambridge CB1 2NZ) which is a Christian-based research and campaigning group formed in 1983 in Cambridge. The main carers project has now moved to Nottingham to continue under the auspices of **The Scripture Union Training Unit** (26-30 Heathcoat Street, Nottingham NG1 3AA). They are concerned with studying and applying Biblical principles to our society. They have already been involved in 'Familybase' a movement to re-emphasise the importance of the family, the 'Keep Sunday Special' Campaign and the 'Freedom from Debt' Campaign. They have been involved in launching a campaign and project concerned with informal care. From their findings they have recently published a handbook called *Serving Carers* which is aimed at helping people within the churches offer practical and other appropriate support at a local level to carers. There is also a video to be used as a companion to the handbook, called *Out of Sight, Out of Mind*. A series of workshops, throughout the country, to draw together people from all denominations, as well as those working in the voluntary and statutory sectors, to discuss what carers in each area need, is also beginning. Another area being explored is the possibility of setting up a Fellowship for Carers - aimed at giving an identity to carers who share the Christian faith. These sound exciting developments both in encouraging the carer and also in informing the Christian church of their needs.

Just as with other voluntary schemes, what the local church or Christian community can offer for the carer will vary very much depending on where you live. But here are some ways in which they may help:

* The clergy, pastors and ministers, and perhaps other members of their congregation, are experienced in counselling and can offer help in this way whether you are a member of their church or not.

* Some churches run schemes for helping needy people in their locality.

* Some run a Good Neighbour scheme (not just for those who attend the church) where someone living locally can drop in on you every so often for company, to check you are alright and perhaps do some simple errands for you.

* The Roman Catholic Church run a scheme which sounds similar called 'St Vincent de Paul'. This was founded by a Frenchman during the French Revolution to help the poor and it has developed from there. Of course neither of these groups is intended solely for carers, and indeed they are probably more concerned with the elderly, lonely and housebound, but no doubt they would be willing to help if they were made aware of your needs.

* In some areas churches are aware of the needs of the carer and have set up groups to help them. For example, in the area where we live (South Lakeland) I have come across one such group who operate on an interdenominational basis to provide a service for carers (as well as the lonely and housebound etc.). They are organised by the Inter Church Council and draw members from all the churches in their town. They provide a relief service (providing sitters etc.) to about 25 people in their locality. People have been referred to them by GPs, social workers, health visitors etc. and are not linked to any church. By reaching out to such people the church is not only supplying practical help but manifesting Christian love and witness.

* Many Christians now recognise the value of Christian counsel, particularly in the area of healing inner hurts, fears and emotional turmoil. Ellel Grange (Ellel, nr. Lancaster LA2 0HN) a centre for Christian healing, counselling and training is one place where people can go to receive healing and wholeness. They have only been running for about four years but are already swamped with enquiries and find it hard to meet the need. Nevertheless, they offer residential healing retreats and counselling sessions to those who require help. They also offer training courses to those involved with, or interested in becoming involved with counselling. Such a place could really meet the needs of a 'hurting' carer and possibly his dependant too. (We have been there and know that the downstairs facilities are suitable for wheelchairs, give or take one or two steps, and that there are ground floor bedrooms).

* Christians also provide marriage counsel. Such weekends or courses are regularly advertised in Christian magazines and your nearest Christian

bookshop might be able to find the details for you. Having said this, these courses are intended for couples and just may not be suitable for a disabled person to attend. Neither might they be intended for people with physical or mental problems. However, it is worth finding out if the facilities are suitable, if you feel such a weekend could help your marriage.

One final comment on all the help available to a carer whether statutory, voluntary or specifically Christian: help will vary considerably depending on the area you live in. Unfortunately it often falls far short of what is needed. This may be because of cut-backs or because of ignorance and indifference. But please, don't despair or give up. Be encouraged by two stories.

Eileen, whose husband suffers from senile dementia was finding it very hard to get any help. Her neighbour, who her husband had often helped in the past and with whom they had been on friendly terms, ceased all contact with the onset of his disease. She would not even bring in a loaf of bread when passing the shop. She received very little help from the health authority or social services either, not even getting replies to her pleas for help. As a result she decided to leave the area completely.

It was quite an upheaval for them both but was obviously the right decision. The social services, nurses, doctor, carers and local villagers have all be 'outstandingly helpful'. She gets regular respite care offered to her husband. Although an agnostic herself, she receives regular visits from a member of the local Housechurch. Her situation has changed completely.

Of course, not everyone is able to take such drastic measures. But if help is not forthcoming try and make your needs known by alerting people to the lack of care in your area. Maybe you can change things. Dorothy has found very little provision in her county. She is writing to her local papers pointing out the lack of statutory and voluntary help. Hopefully things will change for her too.

Chapter 15
RAINBOW'S END

We have a rainbow kitchen. It is basically red and white but it is also filled with rainbows - rainbows painted on a wall, rainbow-coloured ornaments, rainbow pictures - the collection grows! There is a reason behind it.

Several years ago I was talking, in great depth, to a minister about our situation. He prayed for me in a powerful way. As he did so the sky became incredibly dark. We don't get many thunderstorms here but this was a cracker. It was right overhead and I could scarcely see or hear the minister who was right next to me! As he finished praying, the storm began to die down. It was just as if good and evil forces had been fighting it out in the heavens and the good had won! Indeed, as I left he said to me 'Now you don't need to keep dragging this problem to God in prayer anymore. It's all been dealt with just now.'

The circumstances hadn't changed one iota but I felt lighter than I had done for some time. As we came home in the car we had to drive down a steep hill. Our town nestles at the foot of it surrounded by lakeland fells. The view is usually quite spectacular but today it was even more so. Over our town was a magnificent double rainbow. It was as if God was confirming all the minister had said. God had dealt with it all, He was in control and I was to trust Him.

The rainbow is a sign of God's promise. He put it in the sky, after the Flood, to promise Noah and all his descendants for ever afterwards that never again would He bring about such a flood and destruction. The rainbow would serve to remind mankind of this promise. It has now become a symbol of God's promises in general terms - hence my rainbow kitchen! The kitchen declares, in a visual way, the goodness, love and faithfulness of God towards our family. It reminds me to trust Him despite our difficulties.

The kitchen may be a visual reminder of God's love but on its own it would be of little value. It is a useful aid but Chris and I also need to read God's promises in the Bible. We believe the Bible is God's special Word and as such is very powerful. It can actually make a difference to us and have an affect on our lives. It is very worthwhile to actually read and declare (even aloud) what God promises us. It is one thing to 'know' with our heads that God is good, faithful, compassionate etc. but it is another thing to actually 'know' it in our hearts. It isn't always real to us and at those times our circumstances can so easily get on top and we get weighed down with care. But in some strange way, when we read or speak out God's Word it actually becomes real. It is impossible to explain unless you've experienced it for yourself. All I can say is it works. Just try it!

So even if you are still in despair, just be willing to step out and allow God to speak to you and comfort you. It's very hard to take that step. Contrary to popular opinion, Christianity is not a weak option or a prop to hang on to. Yes, it will provide wonderful comfort but it first takes courage and determination to let it take hold of you and affect you.

It really doesn't matter if you don't feel anything or even you don't believe in what you are about to do. Experiment. You have nothing to lose. You can't work faith up by feelings anyway. Faith comes from God. It also comes from hearing God's word (Romans 10:17). So be practical. Take a passage of scripture like Psalm 45 (it speaks of God's compassion and love for all who feel bowed down). Gradually you will actually experience that love for yourself: totally irrational and inexplicable but also totally satisfying. In the same way, when you're feeling anxious, find a passage of scripture which speaks of God's peace and let Him breathe His peace into you and so on!

If you still feel weighed down with despair and doubt and are thinking 'It's alright for her, she has a strong faith. I don't or can't,' then to you I would say 'rubbish!' Chris and I are not special in any way and if we appear to have a strong, unshakeable faith it is because we have dared to allow God into our lives and situation and He has changed us. He has turned our mourning into joy, our fear into peace and filled us with His love and strength.

It is not just our experience either. So many Christians who have written to me have testified to the strength and comfort they (and their dependants) have received from God. Perhaps Jenny, whose mother suffered from senile dementia, sums it all up. Senile dementia must be one of the cruelest afflictions to have to care for. To most of us it appears a horrifying end, completely useless, very distressing and fraught with difficulties. Yet Jenny talks of how her mother's old personality and nature still shone through. She seemed happy and contented even though she could no longer communicate with them and had no idea of her surroundings or what was happening. Her eyes and smile conveyed this. 'God was a great comfort to me and I feel He was a comfort to Mum,' Jenny says. 'She had no need to talk, He knew what her thoughts were and I feel sure He helped her cope and helped us to come to terms with everything.' If God could do that for Jenny's Mum then He can certainly do it for us when we have all our faculties!

We have been taken to the depths of despair and uselessness but I am discovering that as we do proclaim God's wonderful promises to ourselves and others, not only are we restored and feel very whole, well adjusted people, but everything begins to make sense.

We are all precious in God's sight and He has a plan and purpose for each one of us (even a carer and dependant) if only we will accept it. It is not dependent on our circumstances at all. It has to do with knowing and loving Him and wanting to be in His will - wanting to serve and follow Him in the way He wants us to not always as we would want things to be. When we focus on Him and not on ourselves He transcends the circumstances and makes good out of the most dire situation. 'All things work together for good to those that love God ' (Romans 8:28) is true indeed, and Chris and I are only just discovering it!

Even though we've been stripped of doing things that most people take for granted and everything we do manage to do involves that bit more planning and thought, I can honestly say that Chris and I now feel very fulfilled. I'm sure this will remain so as long as we are willing to be in the place God has placed us. This doesn't mean lying down and taking everything that comes and 'meekly' saying 'it's all in the will of God.' Rather, it means getting to know Him better. As we do, we are not only assured of His presence with us and His promises holding true and firm for us, but He will reveal His will to us. God can do this in many ways (but certainly when we pray and read His word, the Bible). All we need do is to simply accept it.

I say 'simply' but accepting God's will for our lives is probably one of the hardest things to do and yet if we don't, it probably accounts for a lot of needless worries and problems which need sorting out. The carer isn't alone in this. However, we need to take that step of faith and accept what we believe to be His will for our lives. When we strive and kick against it or begin doubting whether we have heard right, His presence will elude us. But he doesn't allow us to make mistakes if we are truly in His will and, as we step out, He will reassure us by sending His peace and joy in full measure.

Life can then begin in all its fullness. The end of God's rainbow is never out of our grasp. His promises are as true and unchanging as they were when they were first recorded. They will enable us not only to cope but to triumph. Our lives may never be easy or of our choosing but we can rest in the knowledge that they are in the care of a loving Father and as such will be just right for us and that we are being made into just the kind of people He intended us to be. In His sight we are loved and precious and of great worth.

When I began writing this, I had no idea just how many carers there were and how many other lives were affected too. 'Over a million carers' only refers to those who care for someone in the same household for at least 20 hours a week (although many care for much longer periods). To this number must be added a further five million who care for someone outside their immediate household. They too may be caring for many hours a week on top of having their own homes to run and jobs to go to. Some people may, of course, only be 'caring' for a short time each week. Nevertheless, they will all be faced with some of the problems I have been outlining and will need to seek help and advice.

When one thinks that for every carer there is also a dependant and often other dependants too, it can be seen that caring affects a great number of people. Add to this the number of people who come into contact with a carer (professional, friends, acquaintances and relatives). Viewed in this light, I think it would be true to say that most people will either know a carer or be one themselves or at least have considered becoming one at some point in their lives.

Hopefully, what we have discovered and shared will offer a glimmer of hope to all carers (and where possible their dependants) as well as making others aware of their needs and thus better equipped to deal with them. I hope I have been able to restore a sense of worth and value to those who may appear to be coping magnificently but who deep-down feel confused, frightened, weary, guilty and failing. I hope they will realise they are not alone or abnormal in their emotions and difficulties. I hope they will be encouraged to be brave and step out first towards God and then towards their fellow men to receive all the help and wholeness available to them.

INFORMATION SOURCES

Caring at Home by Nancy Kohner (King's Fund Informal Caring Programme. King's Fund Centre, 126 Albert Street, London NW1 7NF)

Taking a Break (King's Fund Informal Caring Programme)

BBC TV Advice Shop, *Who Cares for You* (supplied by King's Fund Informal Caring Programme)

Carers National Association, 29 Chilworth Mews, London W2 3RG

South Lakeland Council for Voluntary Action ('Caring for the Carers' Project), 102 Highgate, Kendal, Cumbria LA9 4HE

Crossroads Care, 10 Regent Place, Rugby, Warwickshire CV21 2PN

Jubilee Centre, Jubilee House, 3 Hooper Street, Cambridge CB1 2NZ

Christian Council on Ageing, The Old Court, Greens Norton, Nr. Towcester, Northants NN12 8BS

Barnardo's, Tanners Lane, Barkingside, Ilford, Essex IG6 1QG

Cancerlink, 17 Britannia Street, London WC1X 9JN

Ellel Grange, Ellel, nr. Lancaster LA2 0HN

Arthritis News (published by Arthritis Care) - Summer 1990 edition - an article called 'Benefit Changes: Is this really The Way Ahead?' by Jean Ashcroft.

D.S.S. leaflets: FB 2 *Which Benefit?* (April 1990), FB 28 *Sick or Disabled?* (April 1990), NI 212 I.C.A. (April 1990), AB 11 *Help With NHS Costs* (October 1989), NI 211 *Mobility Allowance* (April 1990), NI 205 *Attendance Allowance* (April 1990) and NI 252 S.D.A. (April 1989).